The Medical Interview:

Mastering Skills
for Clinical Practice

The Medical Interview:

Mastering Skills
for Clinical Practice
Third Edition

John L. Coulehan, MD, FACP
Professor of Medicine and Preventive Medicine
State University of New York at Stony Brook
Stony Brook, New York

Marian R. Block, MD, ABFP
Chairperson, Department of Family Medicine
The Western Pennsylvania Hospital
Pittsburgh, Pennsylvania

 F. A. DAVIS COMPANY • Philadephia

F. A. Davis Company
1915 Arch Street
Philadelphia, PA 19103

Printed in the United States of America

Last digit indicates print number: 10 9 8 7 6 5

Senior Medical Editor: Robert W. Reinhardt
Developmental Editor: Bernice M. Wissler
Production Editor: Jessica Howie Martin
Cover Designer: Louis J. Forgione

As new scientific information becomes available through basic and clinical research, recommended treatments and drug therapies undergo changes. The authors and publisher have done everything possible to make this book accurate, up to date, and in accord with accepted standards at the time of publication. The authors, editors, and publisher are not responsible for errors or omissions or for consequences from application of the book, and make no warranty, expressed or implied, in regard to the contents of the book. Any practice described in this book should be applied by the reader in accordance with professional standards of care used in regard to the unique circumstances that may apply in each situation. The reader is advised always to check product information (package inserts) for changes and new information regarding dose and contraindications before administering any drug. Caution is especially urged when using new or infrequently ordered drugs.

Library of Congress Cataloging-in-Publication Data

Coulehan, John L., 1943–
    The medical interview : mastering skill for clinical practice /
John L. Coulehan, Marian R. Block. — Ed. 3.
        p.   cm.
    Includes bibliographical references and index.
    ISBN 0-8036-0267-7 (pbk.)
    1. Medical history taking.   I. Block, Marian R., 1947–
II. Title.
    [DNLM: 1. Medical History Taking.   2. Physician-Patient Relations.
WB 290 CC855m   1997]
RC65.C68   1997
616.07'51—dc 21
DNLM/DLC
for Library of Congress   97-6737
                                                                   CIP

To Our Families

Foreword

• • •

I hesitated in accepting Jack Coulehan and Marian Block's kind invitation to write a foreword for the third edition of their landmark interviewing text. Did I really want to read it for the third time? Since I am the senior editor of a competing text, would I be cutting off my nose to spite my face? Who wants to write a foreword anyway?

On the other hand, a foreword is a chance to put a small frame on a work, to place it into a broader context that may help or inspire the reader. I really enjoyed my reading of the first two editions of their text—it was instructive even for someone like me who is buried in interview research, writing, and organizing. And although the text I edit is suitable for students in the same niche—those starting their journey as clinicians—this text is specifically designed for them and is without equal as a guide to initiate the process.

With that ambivalence on my shoulders, I read through the book as the finished, typeset chapters arrived in small bundles. I was not prepared for the surprise and pleasure I experienced. This is more than just a revision and updating. Every edition of the book has increasingly reflected the authors' love for their work, the growth of their craft as writers, and the development of their special ability to convey difficult concepts in an almost lyrical, certainly inspiring, way. Every edition has taught me a lot.

As a toiler in the vineyards of helping new doctors achieve greater effectiveness, satisfaction, and fascination in this most astonishing profession, I found this book to be like a cold drink under the hot sun. I am so glad the authors have stuck with this project over these many years, since it offers a serious opportunity to students to begin their work with patients with real insight and good habits.

Why is the interview so important and why is it so necessary to teach students about it from the outset of their professional work? The interview is the core clinical skill. It determines the quality and quantity of data the health care professional has to work with in identifying and solving the patient's problems. It determines the quality of the relationship between practitioner (or student practitioner) and patient, a relationship that is key to patient cooperation and satisfaction, to practitioner satisfaction, and to helping the patient grow and develop. It determines as well the patient's understanding of what is going on and being done, his or her willingness to take the risk of a true partnership with the practitioner, and the likelihood that the patient will participate effectively in such matters as going for tests, taking medications, and changing lifestyle.

Surprisingly, most practitioners who are active today have never been observed conducting an interview by someone who is an expert in the process and able to give them feedback. Can you imagine taking a plane in which the pilot had never been observed piloting? Until recent years, most students graduated from medical school and residency without serious curricular commitment to teaching these skills and attitudes, and without real formal knowledge of the rather vast base of data concerning what works and what doesn't. Exaggeration? Just consider the reactions of the public to doctors: they don't listen; they don't understand; they made a mistake because they didn't hear all the facts; they don't care about me, only my money. You have heard these complaints at family gatherings or elsewhere for years. Consider the rates of excess testing, surgery, procedures—all almost 40 to 50 percent higher than in other countries. Consider the rates of detection of mental problems in patients: from 50 to 80 percent of such problems are missed! Consider that doctors as a group are dissatisfied and that studies show that the number one factor in physician job dissatisfaction is the poor quality of doctor-patient relationships.

These are some findings about the importance of the interview and the results of bad training in years past. What do we know about the interview? Approximately 8000 articles, chapters, and monographs have been completed about the interview, and there are at least two quarterly periodicals about it. There are organizations concerned with research and education about it in the United States (The American Academy on Physician and Patient) and the United Kingdom (The Medical Interview Teachers Association). The studies have shown that the interview has three functions: gathering information, developing and maintaining a therapeutic doctor-patient relationship, and educating the patient and negotiating a treatment approach. There are 12 structural elements. Each of these has specific skills that, if performed appropriately, improve the outcomes of the interview process that we care about, such as accuracy and completeness of data. These skills can be taught explicitly and can be measured live or from video review.

We also know something about what succeeds and what fails in teaching these matters. First, knowledge of the interview (its functions and structural elements, why open-ended questions are important, and when such questions should be used), the skills involved (actually practicing each of the elements and types of questions, for example), and the related attitudes ("this is my most important clinical skill; I am going to get it right to begin with and then monitor my effectiveness and continue to grow throughout my professional lifetime") must not only be taught, but must be taught in parallel, in an integrated way. Second, focusing on specific behaviors and practicing with feedback are the best ways to develop good habits, just as in tennis or skiing lessons. Third, attention to the feelings and concerns of the learners as they undergo this major transformation in how they relate to others determines the ultimate outcome. The personal barriers one brings to relationships carry over into the professional arena, and barriers arising from the learning process and from encounters with difficult or traumatic patients can endure and close off critical areas of inquiry or function for the duration of the learner's career.

This book embraces these principles even as it makes the process of learning about the interview entertaining and inspiring. It is like having the opportunity to learn to dance from Balanchine or to play tennis from Arthur Ashe. Placing your future in the sure hands of Coulehan and Block is a wise move that will help to ensure a strong start on your journey.

MACK LIPKIN, JR., MD
NEW YORK

Acknowledgments

• • •

T*he Medical Interview* includes numerous examples of physician-patient interactions. Almost all are abstracted from taped interviews, although in every case we have removed personal references that might serve to identify the physician or patient. In some cases we have altered the transcripts (mostly by shortening) in ways that serve to demonstrate specific points more compactly. We are grateful to the patients and physicians who permitted us to tape and publish these conversations.

We wish also to acknowledge our debt to teachers and colleagues. Three outstanding physician-educators deserve special thanks. Eric J. Cassell, MD, taught us how to observe the physician-patient interaction systematically and encouraged us in this work for many years. Alvan Feinstein, MD, taught us that the medical interview is a source of scientific data about the patient and inspired us to find the science in the art of history taking. Kenneth D. Rogers, MD, gave us the wholehearted and sustained support we needed, first, to develop our course in medical interviewing and, later, to write this book.

In the years since the first edition of this book was published, we have continued to learn from our students, our patients, and our colleagues, as well as from the burgeoning literature on the analysis of physician-patient interactions. We also want to thank Marcy Cloherty and Lisa Dougherty, who provided invaluable help in preparing the manuscript and coordinating the endless mail, fax, and telephone interactions of two authors now working in offices 500 miles apart.

Although each of us had primary responsibilities for writing certain chapters, this book is a joint product; in a very special sense it is truly a collaborative effort, and we are both responsible for the entire text.

John L. Coulehan, MD, FACP
Marian R. Block, MD, ABFP

Contents

• • •

Introduction

• • •

THE POOR HISTORIAN

History-taking, the most clinically sophisticated procedure of medicine, is an extraordinary investigative technique: in few other forms of scientific research does the observed object talk.

Alvan Feinstein

Clinical Judgment

They cluster in the hall on rounds, eight of them—students, house officers, and attending physician—creating turbulence and obstructing flow. A medication nurse pushes a cabinet around them on the way down the hall, while the breakfast lorry closes in from the other direction. An intern begins the presentation with "Mr. Blank is a 52-year-old man who presents with abdominal pain . . . the patient is a poor historian. . . ."

The attending physician learns that this sick person "claims" to have a number of symptoms and is apparently taking several medications. The intern hastens to add that Mr. Blank's compliance is poor; he doesn't seem to understand his illness; and he is, after all, a "poor historian." Having thus dispensed with preliminaries, the intern moves on to reporting the patient's physical findings and initial laboratory data. At this point all qualifiers are dropped: the magnesium level does not *seem* to be 2.2, it *is* 2.2. Meanwhile, the attending physician reflects on the term "poor historian," perhaps because of an unconscionable lack of interest in magnesium. The matrix of numbers vibrating among students and house officers takes on a life of its own while the attending physician wonders about this patient's "poorness."

The physician knows what the intern is trying to tell the group with the phrase "poor historian." The young physician does not intend to say that the patient is an impoverished professor of history. Nor does he or she mean that the patient is a history student with poor grades. No, the intern is saying in precise medical shorthand, "I was unable to reconstruct a logical story of the illness in my conversation with this patient. We did not communicate well." Reflecting further, the attending physician finds the term "poor historian" acceptable but wonders if the attribution is correct. Perhaps the intern would be more correct in saying, "The medical history is unclear because *I'm* a poor historian."

This vignette illustrates how data we obtain from speaking with the patient and the therapy we accomplish through the process of physician-patient interaction are not often topics for discussion during medical rounds. Although we consider information about serum magnesium, for which accuracy and precision is assumed, a fit topic for discussion, knowledge of the precise pattern of symptoms or the patient's beliefs about the symptoms appears less scientific and less relevant. Clinical students soon learn to spend less time listening to the patient's story and more time among their peers at the unit station agonizing over the meaning of a magnesium value. Trainees learn to accept responsibility for how well (or how poorly) they perform a bone marrow aspiration, interpret an x-ray, or insert a flexible sigmoidoscope. As physicians, we rarely blame the patient for an inadequate bone marrow aspirate, yet we believe the hospital is full of patients who perpetrate poor histories.

Stories of sickness and suffering—the kind of human stories that moved us to enter a healing profession in the first place—gradually move to the background as we become "socialized" into the technical culture of medicine. Students and physicians become preoccupied with quite different stories, technical tales in which organs and instruments rather than people are the protagonists. Sometimes, in fact, the patient's story is entirely forgotten: nowadays it is not rare in clinical practice for investigations to bring some unexpected results to light, and these lead to more examinations along a side track. After a while the whole staff is interested in, say, the incidental finding of a renal cyst on an abdominal CT scan, and nobody remembers why the patient was admitted. Only on the day the patient is discharged will he or she complain, "But you haven't done anything about my fatigue!"

This illustrates a narrow view of the clinical enterprise, one that permeates medical education; the view is that real medicine is solely concerned with objective data such as numbers, graphs, and images. This is associated with the belief that so-called subjective data (for example, the story a patient tells us) are necessarily lacking in quantification and so also must be lacking in clinical value. In other words, what patients feel, the suffering they experience, and the disability that haunts them, all of which they describe only indirectly through the medium of words, are secondary in importance to those physiologic quantities that can be observed directly by physicians. Physicians, according to this premise, must address what causes all this suffering and pain: altered physiology, abnormal biochemical findings, or disease. The real work of medicine requires us to reduce persons and their illnesses to organs and diseases. In this view, if you correct bad numbers, suffering will go away. You don't have to pay much attention to who the patients are or to the fine details of their stories.

In fact, the patient and his or her story often get in the way of "real" medicine. The patient "comes to function as a kind of translucent screen on which the disease is projected . . . (but) the screen has opacities of its own which obscure the accurate perception of the underlying disease."[1] The poor historian, the patient with whom we have difficulty communicating, has many such "opacities." It is difficult to see through the person to observe the disease.

But should the patient be merely an obstructive screen that we try to work around or to see through? A broader view of medicine holds that the patient's stories—stories of sickness—lie at the center of medical practice. The great clinician and medical educator William Osler wrote, "It is a safe rule to have no teaching without a patient for a text, and the best teaching is that taught by the patient himself." In fact, experienced clinicians are aware that, in general, about 70 percent of diagnoses are made on the basis of patient interviews and over 90 percent are made on the basis of history and physical examination. Primary physicians spend the largest part of their clinical time talking with patients; they generate most of their diagnostic hypotheses on the basis of the history, and most of the significant bits of information they use arise from this dialogue.

Despite widespread lip-service to this broader view of medicine, until the last 20 years medical schools generally did not include interviewing skills in their curricula. Medical educators did not consider history taking and talking with patients appropriate topics for serious study. These educators gave students "little black books" that included lists of questions about symptoms and past diagnoses. If the patient did not answer these questions clearly, concisely, and in a medically acceptable fashion, the patient was labeled a "poor historian." Clinicians told their students, "Talking with patients is important, but you'll pick up how to do it as you go along. The doctor-patient relationship is also important—crucial, in fact—but you'll pick that up as you go along, too. You just need experience."

For a number of reasons, this attitude toward communication skills in medicine has changed in recent years. First, we have discovered that highly specialized, machine-intensive medicine is not necessarily the "best" medicine. Patients often find themselves doing better by the numbers but feeling worse. They may undergo the most advanced tests and see the "best" specialists, but find themselves feeling just as sick, and often angry and confused as well. At the same time, academic physicians have begun to understand that pain, suffering, and dysfunction must be conceptualized in broad human terms as well as in biochemical terms if we are to be effective healers. Clinical practice must be based on a biopsychosocial or holistic model rather than on a purely biologic model.

Second, in the last generation more and more investigators have studied the process of interviewing and analyzed its individual components. This work, along with studies in fields as wide-ranging as medical anthropology and clinical decision making, has shown that the "art of medicine" can be articulated and taught systematically. It is not simply a matter of intuition and experience.

Third, patient-oriented studies have shown that good patient-physician communication leads to good outcomes, improved patient satisfaction, and better adherence to treatment. Alternatively, poor patient-physician communication leads to poor outcomes, doctor-shopping, and excessive malpractice suits. In fact, when an adverse event occurs, physician insensitivity and poor communication are the major factors in a patient's decision to sue.[2,3] Finally, the pressing need to limit the costs of medical care has led to a renewed emphasis on generalist care, in which physicians use resources more rationally by knowing more about their patients. This certainly has been a key feature in the movement toward HMOs and other managed-care arrangements.

This book is based on the premise that interviewing and patient-physician communication are essential to good medical practice. Talking with patients is not a skill reserved for psychiatrists and primary care doctors. It is essential for radiologists as well as internists, ophthalmologists as well as pediatricians. Medical interviewing is a basic clinical skill. It is not a matter of common sense, nor does it come necessarily with experience. It is a skill that can be broken down into its component parts, and it can be learned. That is the subject of this book.

The Medical Interview is addressed primarily to students of medicine and other health professions who are about to begin their professional interaction with patients. It is designed to be a guide for those who are just learning to take a medical history and interact with patients, as well as a resource for those who are further along in their education, including postgraduate trainees. Our particular emphasis is on the microskills of the initial patient interview. Although we deal extensively with basic history taking, the same skills serve as building blocks for all types of patient-physician interactions. They lie at the core of the art and science of medicine.

The book is divided into two major sections. *Basic Skills: Understanding the Patient's Story* presents fundamentals of clinical interviewing (Chaps. 1 and 2) and various components of the medical history (Chaps. 3 through 7). *Basic Skills in Practice: Applying the Patient's Story* deals with more complex or difficult interviewing situations, along with additional topics relevant to the clinical interview. Chapters 8 and 9 consider aspects of the interview as adapted to pediatric, geriatric, primary-care, and managed-care encounters. We review various barriers to communication and sensitive or difficult situations in Chapters 10 and 11. The final chapters deal with screening and case finding through the use of questionnaires (Chap. 12), clinical judgment as manifested in patient-physician conversations (Chap. 13), understanding the patient's beliefs and values (Chap. 14), and patient education and negotiation (Chap. 15).

References

1. Baron RJ. Bridging clinical distance: An empathic rediscovery of the known. *J Med Philosophy* 1981; 6:5.
2. Beckman HB, Markakis KM, Suchman L, Frankel RM. The doctor-patient relationship and malpractice. Lessons from plaintiff depositions. *Arch Intern Med* 1994; 154:1365–1370.
3. Vincent C, Young M, Phillips A. Why do people sue doctors? A study of patients and relatives taking legal action. *The Lancet* 1994; 343:1609–1613.

Suggested Readings

Hunter KM. *Doctor's Stories. The Narrative Structure of Medical Knowledge.* Princeton, NJ, Princeton University Press, 1991.

Lipkin M Jr., Putnam S, Lazare A. *The Medical Interview: Clinical Care, Education, and Research.* New York, Springer-Verlag, 1995.

PART ONE

BASIC SKILLS: UNDERSTANDING THE PATIENT'S STORY

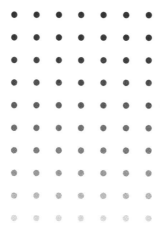

CHAPTER 1

I Attach the Same Meaning

• • •

INTERVIEWING AS A CLINICAL SKILL

A very good way to find out how another person is thinking or feeling is to ask him . . . At this point, however, a difficulty arises. If I am to acquire information in this way about another person's experiences, I must understand what he says about them. And this would seem to imply that I attach the same meaning to his words as he does. But how, it may be asked, can I ever be sure that this is so?

A. J. Ayer, *The Problem of Knowledge*

Although medicine is based on a group of theoretical sciences, clinical medicine itself is a practical science: it is the science of helping ill people get well, rather than that of understanding disease. Like any other science, clinical medicine has basic units of observation, basic quantities of measurement, and basic instruments for obtaining these measurements. The units of observation are signs and symptoms, the quantities of measurement are words and sometimes numbers, and the most important instrument is the medical practitioner.[1] Like any other scientific instrument, the clinician must be objective, precise, sensitive, specific, and reliable when making observations about the patient's illness. In this text we examine interviewing and interactional skills as fundamental to the science of medicine. As we will show, interviewing skills are also at the core of the art of medicine. In fact, in medicine, art and science are synergistic.

OBJECTIVITY

What does it mean to be objective when interviewing a patient and taking a medical history? **Objectivity** means striving to remove one's own beliefs, prejudices, and preconceptions from observations; it involves eliminating bias or systematic distortion from one's observations. Other words for objectivity are **accuracy** and **validity**. The illness data should correspond to what the patient really felt and experienced. If, for example, you start with a preconceived notion of the illness and you discard or minimize ill-fitting items, you are not being objective. Consider this interview taken from an article by Platt and McMath.[1] The physician here "knows" that the patient has severe lung disease and so is unable to hear the chief complaint:

Dr: Hello, I'm Dr. X, are you Mrs. Y?

Pt: Yes, I'm glad to know you.

Dr: What sorts of troubles have you been having?

Pt: I've been going downhill for 2 years. Nothing seems to be working right.

Dr: What is the worst part?

Pt: My legs. I have constant pain in my legs. It's gotten so bad I can't sleep.

Dr: What about your breathing?

Pt: Oh, that's all right. I can breathe fine. I just hurt so bad in my legs.

Dr: Are you still smoking?

Pt: Yes, with this pain, I've gone back to cigarettes for relief. But I'm down to half a pack or so a day.

Dr: Are you having pains in your chest?

Pt: No.

Dr: How about cough?

Pt: No, I hardly ever cough.

Dr: How much are you actually able to do?

Pt: Well, I was able to do everything until about 2 years ago, but now I can hardly walk half a block.

Dr: Why is that?

Pt: My legs. They hurt.

Dr: Do they swell up?

Pt: Well, they've been a bit swollen the last 2 or 3 weeks, but the pain is there whether they swell or not.

Dr: All right, I want to ask you some things about your medical history now.

The physician in this case seems to ignore the patient's leg pain; when she complains about it, the physician replies with questions about breathing. The clinician is undervaluing certain kinds of information—what he doesn't expect—while overvaluing data related to a diagnosis that he "knows," namely the patient's chronic lung disease. Failure of objectivity is unscientific and could lead to a missed diagnosis; it is also likely to make the patient feel ignored. When patients feel ignored, they tend to say less, and opportunities to obtain other important data may be lost.

How might the same physician respond on a better day?

Dr: Hello, I'm Dr. X, are you Mrs. Y?

Pt: Yes, I'm glad to know you.

Dr: Thank you, I'm glad to know you too. What sorts of troubles have you been having?

Pt: I've been going downhill for 2 years. Nothing seems to be working right.

Dr: What is the worst part?

Pt: My legs. I have constant pain in my legs. It's gotten so bad I can't sleep.

Dr: Pain in your legs. Tell me more about that.

Pt: Well, it's gotten so bad I can hardly walk half a block.

Dr: You mean the pain forces you to stop?

Pt: Yes, that's exactly it. And, well, it gets better when I stop, but never really goes away. Even at night when I'm lying still it wakes me up, it's so bad.

The patient now is describing claudication, a symptom characteristic of severe peripheral vascular disease. The patient is now able to volunteer important details about the leg pain that not only aid the diagnostic process but also help her feel understood. **The skill in being objective requires, first, effective listening and, then, effective feedback to the patient of what you have heard; in other words, you let the patient know that you understand.**

INTERPRETATION VERSUS OBSERVATION

It is easy to confuse interpretation with observation. When talking with a patient, your observation is what the patient actually says or does; the patient's words are primary data. Students are sometimes encouraged by preceptors and house officers to use terms that are really interpretations rather than descriptions. One example of such a term is "claudication," as in our example here; another is "angina," a certain kind of chest pain caused by coronary artery disease. These words are interpretations because they imply specific etiologies. The primary data of the symptom "angina" might be something like: "substernal discomfort of a dull, pressing nature, lasting about 3 minutes, brought on by exertion, and relieved by rest." Interpretive terms are a shorthand necessary for thinking and conversation in medicine; such terms are appropriate when the symptom has indeed been shown to be, as in this case, secondary to coronary artery disease. However, if you interpret the symptom prematurely, once you start using the word "angina," you may forget the patient's story and ignore data that point to the correct diagnosis. **Premature interpretation compromises objectivity.**

For example, here is a 68-year-old woman who lived for several years with the diagnosis of angina—that is, coronary artery disease—because her physician did not "hear" the primary data. Here is how she described her chest pain:

Dr: Tell me about this chest pain.

Pt: It's a soreness in here, right through here (pointing to midchest) a lot. Some pain in my arm and a feeling here. And a burning in the middle here and a burning in my throat.

Dr: When does this pain seem to come on?

Pt: Oh, it can be any time, doctor. Sometimes I even get it in the middle of the night.

Dr: How about when you walk or are active in any way?

Pt: No, I can just be sitting.

Despite the fact that the patient did not have and had never had exertional chest pain relieved by rest, she had a complete cardiac workup, including coronary angiography. Even though the test results proved negative, she carried a diagnosis of coronary artery disease and lived a confined and limited lifestyle due to fear. Finally, a new physician heard the story of burning and the nocturnal occurrence of pain and ordered an esophagram and upper gastrointestinal series, which revealed massive esophageal reflux and spasm. Perhaps it would have been more serious to overlook coronary artery disease, but for the patient much was lost. Frightened that she might die at any moment of a heart attack, she persisted in her belief that she had heart disease and was unable to be rehabilitated to an active life.

Objectivity means avoiding premature interpretation on your part; it also means distinguishing between the primary data and the patient's interpretation of what it means. This is important to remember when a patient tells you, "My ulcer is acting up," or "My heart is giving me a lot of trouble," or "I'm here for my Hodgkin's disease." In such instances, the patient is interpreting certain symptoms as indicative of the presence of peptic ulcer or other known disease.

Here, for example, is the statement of a 78-year-old man who called his physician with the following complaint:

Pt: I don't know what's wrong. Somebody said I must have had the flu but it's lasted so long and I've tried everything and I don't know what to eat, so I just had to call and find out what you thought because it's been going on now 2 weeks and—you know me—I don't call unless I really have to. And someone said I must have appendicitis or what's that thing that old people get?

This patient focuses on the etiology of his problem and does not tell the story of his symptoms. All we know is that, whatever has been going on, it has been going on for about 2 weeks and is probably related to the GI tract. The physician's next response might be:

Dr: Well, some people who get the flu do feel sick for quite some time.

Although this response shows that the physician has heard the patient's theory, the physician still would not know what is going on. A better response might be:

Dr: Well, some people who get the flu do feel sick for quite a while, but I'm not sure you had the flu. What exactly were your symptoms?
Pt: Well, I had severe diarrhea—just like water—for a few days and I hurt low down in my belly. And weak, awful weak.

The doctor now has some primary data with which to start putting the diagnostic puzzle together.

Although the patient's interpretation should be considered separately from symptom data, the interpretation should not be ignored; it is important to acknowledge his belief about etiology as legitimate, whether or not you agree with it. Such recognition of the patient's point of view is necessary in a therapeutic relationship and will maximize your opportunities for patient engagement and education (see Chap. 15). In this case, the physician might well explain why the patient's appendicitis theory is unlikely, rather than simply ignoring it.

PRECISION

Precision is a characteristic of the scientific process that relates to the distribution of observations around the "real" value. Precise observations cluster around the mean, whereas imprecise observations are widely scattered. The basic units of measurement in a medical interview are words. In a medical history, words describe sensations perceived by the patient and communicated to the clinician. As verbal measurements, words should be precise. They should be sufficiently detailed and unambiguous to indicate the "real" data.

In the issue of precision we are dealing not with a systematic bias that leads purposefully in one direction or another, but rather with random, unsystematic error introduced by vagueness, poor listening, or lack of attention to detail. For example, if a patient complains of being tired, does "tired" mean that the patient has shortness of breath, muscle weakness, lack of desire for activity, or sleepiness? Although the clinician may correctly register the patient's words, he or she may have no idea what is actually being described unless there is sufficient detail to distinguish among dyspnea, muscle weakness, lack of motivation, and somnolence. To make this distinction, the next question might go something like, "What do you mean by tired?" or "Can you tell me more about this tiredness?" or "How would you describe this feeling without using the word 'tired'?" The good interviewer attempts to discover as precisely as possible what the patient is actually experiencing.

Here is an example of a physician trying to get a precise history about the patient's chief complaint of headache:

Pt: See, I get these migraine headaches.

Dr: What do you mean by migraine headaches?

Pt: The last two headaches—I had two headaches last week, one on Monday and one on Thursday. Now they weren't real, real bad but the ones that I had before that, I threw up. I got real, real cold.

Dr: How often do you get these headaches?

Pt: I had two real bad ones within 2 weeks' time, then I didn't have one for a few weeks. Now the ones that I had last week, I didn't throw up with them, but they were enough that I had to go to bed with them.

Dr: Are the headaches something that occur almost every week, almost every month, or every couple of months?

Pt: I get them all the time. It is just within the last few months that I have been getting them more frequently. But I have averaged maybe one or two a month.

Dr: When you get these headaches, where does it hurt?

Pt: They start here and they just go around (demonstrating on his head). Sometimes they'll go on one side of my face, sometimes on the other side of my face. But they start in the back of my neck here.

Dr: Do you get any kind of problems with your eyes when these headaches are coming on?

Pt: Blurred vision. The light bothers me.

Dr: Both eyes or one eye?

Pt: I have to go, like, I go upstairs in my bedroom and like close everything up, and I just lay down with a blanket.

Dr: What kind of problem does the light give you when you have a headache?

Pt: It just bothers me, just the light itself, it's like a glare. The light itself bothers me.

Dr: What do these headaches keep you from doing?

Pt: Everything. I can't do a thing. When I get one, I have to go to bed. That's exactly what I do. Usually I throw up with them. I get real, real cold. It can be 90 degrees outside, I'm freezing. Mostly the throwing up is a light vomiting.

Dr: Is there anything you can think of that triggers these headaches?

Pt: Nothing, it just starts.

Dr: Okay. What kind of person are you?

Pt: Little things will set me off. Like my kids are fighting, that bothers me, or if I feel like I'm overly tired or something like that. Little things bother me, that's all, but I've always been a nervous person.

Dr: When you get upset or you get nervous, is that likely to start up your headaches? Is there any kind of connection between the two?

Pt: I can get up with a headache. If I get up with it, I'm done for the whole day. I do nothing at all.

Dr: Do these headaches scare you?

Pt: No, I'm used to them.

Dr: Okay, so they don't frighten you, it's just a matter of trying to . . .

Pt: To get rid of them.

There is no unambiguous test for the etiology of headache; only a careful and precise history can distinguish between migraine and muscle contraction headaches. By asking, "What do you mean by migraine headache?," this physician does not accept the patient's or previous doctor's diagnosis of "migraine" (an interpretation) and goes on to get many details (precision) about frequency, location, visual symptoms, and other associated symptoms.

SENSITIVITY AND SPECIFICITY

Accuracy and precision are two criteria by which we judge medical data, including the medical history. Two additional criteria are **sensitivity** and **specificity**. The sensitivity of a test expresses its ability to "pick up" real cases of the disease in question. The higher the sensitivity, the greater the percentage of cases identified accurately by the test as being cases. Specificity, on the other hand, refers to a test's ability to "rule out" disease in normal people. The higher the specificity, the greater the likelihood that a negative test result actually identifies a person who does not have the disease. Few, if any, tests in medicine approach 100 percent sensitivity and specificity; certainly the medical interview will not yield such definitive information.

A symptom may be very sensitive (most people with pneumonia have cough) but not specific at all (dozens of diseases cause cough); it may be relatively specific (nocturnal midepigastric pain relieved by eating in cases of duodenal ulcer) but not very sensitive (most persons with duodenal ulcer do not have that symptom). This relative lack of sensitivity and specificity for individual symptoms is one reason why physicians often minimize the value of history taking and rush into more "scientific" tests. However, an individual symptom is rarely the appropriate unit upon which to base decisions; we deal, rather, with symptom complexes, patterns, or stories. We consider a detailed reconstruction of the illness, rather than isolated statements about symptoms—not just one symptom, but many; not just one point in time, but the whole story.

A complete symptom complex may well be quite sensitive and specific; it may be adequate, in fact, to serve as the basis for diagnosis and therapy. Even when the "complete" history does not contain enough information for a correct diagnosis, the history usually contains *most* of the needed information. Moreover, the history narrows the range of possible problems dramatically and yields a very small number of hypotheses to be ruled out, supported, or confirmed by physical examination and further studies. Thus, even in high-technology settings, such as university training programs, residents generally regard the medical history as having greater diagnostic value than either physical examination or laboratory and radiographic tests.[2] The well-conducted patient interview will yield a firm (and large) database on which to design an efficient (and small) diagnostic plan. To achieve this result, however, the physician must approach the task objectively and precisely. The real sensitivity and specificity of a symptom complex are irrelevant in a given situation if the instrument through which the data are obtained—you, the clinician—lacks accuracy and precision.

REPRODUCIBILITY

Reproducibility or **reliability** is another important characteristic of scientific tests, including medical interviewing. Different observers should be able to obtain the same results. In the medical history, however, reproducibility must be tempered by several considerations about human nature and the interactive process. In caring for a patient in the hospital, three or four observers are likely to obtain three or four different versions of the patient's story. Much of the time, the differences may not be of great significance, but sometimes they will be crucial. Only one of four observers, for example, may note that the patient has had bright red rectal bleeding intermittently for the last 3 months. This fact might be lost in the review of systems because the patient actually came into the hospital for chest pain and was either too embarrassed to mention the bleeding or, perhaps, too concerned about his heart to mention a seemingly unrelated problem. It suddenly becomes an important issue when you find the patient has a stool guaiac test result that demonstrates occult blood or a hematocrit value of 32 percent. The medical team might have to shift gears from an ischemic heart disease workup to a lower GI bleeding workup. Of course, just as in the laboratory, data that change from one "experiment" to the next are suspect. Reproducibility is a characteristic highly valued in testing; this apparent lack of reproducibility makes many physicians question the value of medical history taking.

There are several reasons why various observers may get varying stories at different times.

First, every patient comes to the hospital or to the doctor with a personal story that includes a series of symptoms, but most patients have no benchmark indicating which of these are more or less important in explaining their underlying disease. A severe headache may cause more pain than a sudden swelling of the left leg, but the latter could be secondary to lymphatic obstruction by metastatic cancer, whereas the former may have no pathologic significance at all. Each time a person is interviewed and is asked to construct his or her story, the person learns, by virtue of the questions asked, what is of most importance to the interviewer. The patient learns, in a sense, to "package" the story and make it more efficient or relevant or interesting to the clinician. Therefore, it is likely that later observers will get a more clearly connected and flowing—and certainly different—history than the first interviewer.

Second, a corollary to this "educational" process is that patients may learn to consider important some things that they had not bothered to mention originally. The person may have forgotten the first episode of syncope or considered an illness that occurred 3 years earlier to be entirely unrelated to the current illness. Repetition and focusing on specific symptoms not only will make the story more coherent but will also refresh the patient's memory or, perhaps, set the stage for some new insight. Therefore, it is reasonable to assume that later observers may pick up entirely new information that the patient neglected to mention earlier.

For example, here is how a first interview might go with a patient complaining of headaches. Knowing the importance to the diagnosis of differentiating new headaches from chronic ones, the clinician, a student, proceeds:

Dr: Tell me about your headaches. When did they start?

Pt: Well, I started getting them about 3 months ago.

Dr: Is that the first time you ever had this headache?

Pt: Well, yes.

Dr: So headaches are really new for you.

Pt: Well, now that I think about it, I can remember one something like it about 2 years ago. I remember, we were on vacation and I had to stay in the hotel. I thought I had the flu or something.

Dr: That's interesting. When did you get the next one?

For the next clinician, the attending physician, who interviews this patient, the story may be revealed as follows:

Dr: Tell me when these headaches started.

Pt: Well, I guess the first time I ever had one was about 2 years ago. But then I only had one every few months or so; they weren't frequent until about 3 months ago when I started getting them every week.

Although both interviewers ask similar questions, notice how the patient's story is more organized and straightforward on the second telling. The first interviewer had to "dig" harder for the onset 2 years ago and could have missed it entirely.

Third, sick people may have already "organized" their illness in some way that makes sense to them before they see the doctor.[3] They may have tried getting rid of the symptoms on their own and perhaps may have asked for advice from family or friends. They may have read health columns in newspapers or seen a "TV doctor" discussing a problem similar to theirs. In addition, some patients may have religious or cultural beliefs that "frame" their understanding of illness in general and their own symptoms in particular (see Chap. 14). In these ways, patients usually develop hypotheses or reasons for their problems and have ideas about what can or should be done about them. Consequently, they are likely to tell their stories in ways consistent with these hypotheses; they will emphasize symptoms that support their theories and minimize or forget symptoms that do not. The primary data—perceived symptoms—are filtered through the patient's own beliefs. In the process of being interviewed by several different people focusing on medical hypotheses, a patient's own hypotheses about the data may change. And when the story is filtered through a different set of beliefs, the story's elements—perceptions, symptoms, and attributions—appear to change.

Fourth, different histories may be obtained at different times because the patient simply and consciously changes the story. Clinicians often invoke this reason when they dislike the patient or are unable to account for the symptoms. The more the symptoms seem to be unrelated to "objective" findings or diagnostic tests, the more likely they are to be considered exaggerated or even imaginary and, therefore, susceptible to change from one history-taking session to another. Although some patients, of course, do change their stories, the so-called unreliable patient is a much less frequent explanation for apparent inconsistences than the other factors we are considering.

Fifth, interviewing skills play a part as well. An empathic physician who lets the patient tell his or her story is much more likely to obtain an accurate picture than a physician who asks a list of questions by rote. Interviewing expertise probably bears a general relationship to the person's experience level (student, postgraduate trainee, practicing clinician), but when one considers an individual interview of an individual patient, all bets are off. The inexperienced student who is able to spend time with a patient in a non-threatening atmosphere may learn a lot more than a hurried attending physician. **In general, interviewing skills that maximize objectivity and precision produce more accurate data and reduce the rate of false-positive (making a diagnosis that isn't there) and false-negative (missing the diagnosis) histories.**

SCIENCE AND ART AT WORK

As you develop clinical skills, you learn techniques to achieve objectivity and precision in gathering primary data from patients (Fig. 1–1, page 14). These skills make good science and, what is more, allow the patient to "connect" with you in a therapeutic relationship. Thus, the basic skills of interviewing as an **art** serve also as pre-conditions for the **scientific** collection and analysis of clinical data. **Throughout this book you will find that our emphasis is on the interdependence of science and art in clinical practice.**

Is there a contradiction between a "just get the facts" interview and an empathic interview? There is no such contradiction; you cannot get the facts without "understanding exactly" (Carl Rogers' definition of empathy[4]) and without suspending judgment. Otherwise, the "facts" that you get may be irrelevant, or worse, untrue. With such an approach, you will embark on a vicious cycle that leads you to undervalue interviewing, and rely less and less

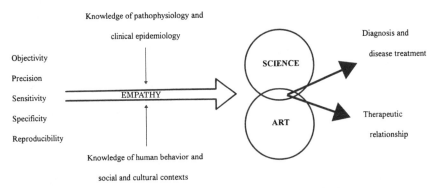

FIGURE 1–1. The art and science of medical interviewing.

on listening to the patient. To get the facts, you must understand and not judge; if you do otherwise, you will lose primary data essential to making a correct diagnosis. And when you understand and are nonjudgmental, you will build rapport—often the start of a therapeutic relationship—and you will gather the data that tell not only *what* the diagnosis is but *who* the patient is.

A patient says this best. The following is part of an interview in which the patient describes how it feels to be understood and not judged:

Pt: Aw, I'm not usually this able to talk to people like this. I don't really know you. . . .

Dr: That's true. I'm a total stranger.

Pt: And all of a sudden I have gone completely down the line and told you everything I could possibly think of to tell you. I've never been able to do that. I have very few people that I talk to personally or talk to about the way I feel . . um . . I talk to my family but there are only certain things that you can talk to your family about, and I have never had anyone I could talk to. I have always kept everything to myself. And now, all of a sudden, I've just flowed over like a broken toilet.

Dr: Was it helpful?

Pt: Yes, because I just learned something else about myself. The funny thing is, I have said all these things to you, and most times talking to people, I always think before I talk. I have said everything I have said to you without thinking about it first, and without wondering what you are going to think about what I am saying to you. And I can honestly say that I have never done that with anyone.

Dr: Uh huh.

Pt: I . . um . . have, maybe, I have a lot of friends but I mean, people you can really sit down and tell every little thing that happens in your life.

There are very few of those. And I even, I even think before I say what I say to them because there's always a chance that someone misinterprets, and really deep down I always know I want their opinion because I know they are my friends, and they are going to say what I want to hear and that's not always what I need to hear.

Dr: Well, I'm glad. Because I like to think it's helpful.

Pt: It really is. I feel quite good about the whole thing.

The patient here describes being able to say everything "without thinking about it first." He is describing his ability to reveal uncensored data that are vital to the diagnostic process; he was able to do this because he wasn't "wondering what you are going to think about what I am saying to you." This is precisely the aim of competent medical history taking. Revealing uncensored data was crucial for this patient, who presented with a rash that proved to be secondary syphilis acquired in the course of multiple homosexual contacts. Had he filtered out the story of his sexual activity, about which he was embarrassed and ambivalent, the diagnosis would have been made less quickly or, perhaps, not at all. He later died of AIDS, and the need to communicate openly remained vital to his care.

SAGA OF THE FIFTH WHEEL

This section is an aside to address certain concerns of students who are just beginning to learn patient interviewing and physical examination. It is perhaps inevitable that the beginning student sometimes feels like a spare part or a "fifth wheel." He or she has little or no responsibility for patient care. The patients may be sick, fatigued, and disgruntled at having to interact with a student. Besides simple inexperience and the anxiety associated with it, this situation leads students to have several other realistic concerns about their first interviews. Three of the major ones are:

- I don't know enough about pathophysiology to do a good history and physical examination, let alone to "get" the diagnosis.
- The patients have been worked over 10 times already and are generally tired of it all, and sometimes angry, by the time I come in to examine them.
- I have no responsibility for the patient, nor the ability to help, so I feel like an interloper—a fifth wheel.

Of course, each of these statements has an element of truth, but none of them need be a major constraint in your interviewing and physical diagnosis experience. Let us deal with each concern.

First, "I don't know enough pathophysiology." It is clear that you are not going to characterize patterns of symptoms as efficiently as an experienced physician, nor will you be able to pick up subtle physical signs. You might, for example, examine a patient with peptic ulcer disease before you study the GI tract in your pathophysiology course. You will complain, "I don't know what symptoms to ask about. I don't know what direction to take." As long as the content of the history (or physical examination) is all that interests you, there is no way to get beyond your lack of knowledge. However, the clinical art (and the point of this book) is to learn the process and method. Your goal is to learn to talk with patients in a way that maximizes both information gathering and therapeutic communication. The diagnosis (although interesting) is largely irrelevant at this point—you are not expected to make good diagnostic hypotheses without a knowledge of relevant pathophysiology. Your goal is to characterize the symptoms and the person as precisely and objectively as possible and, more importantly, to create an interview situation in which this can occur. Unfortunately, some studies have suggested that the interviewing skills of medical students actually decline as they progress from their first to their fourth year and learn more about disease.[5,6]

Second, "The patients have often had many other examinations and are sick and tired of it all." The anger your patient expresses (or just barely conceals) very frequently arises not from the mere fact of repeated examinations, but from the whole situation—being ill, having a backache that no one pays attention to, uncomfortable diagnostic studies, doctors who are rude or preoccupied, nurses who seem unsympathetic, and so forth. The anger is present even before you arrive on the scene.

How do you deal with this? It is crucial to clarify your role, not just as a student, but as a student learning to do an interview—someone who will not be taking care of the patient on the hospital unit. Then, make sure the patient has really consented to your interview and examination with a comment or question, such as "May I talk with you now about the problems that brought you to the hospital?" If he or she does not wish to talk with you and says so, let it go at that. For patients who are tired or in pain, suggest the possibility of your coming in later. If the patient seems angry, acknowledge the anger. This will give you a good opportunity to see how effective "interchangeable" responses can be (see "Levels of Responding" in Chap. 2) in obtaining information and developing rapport.

Sick people, like anyone else, may have several mutually conflicting feelings at the same time. A given patient may want to be helpful to a student but simultaneously be angry about the situation, depressed about being ill, and simply exhausted. You can tip the balance in your favor: By being honest with the patient and really listening, you will avoid contributing to the patient's anger and will also tend to defuse it.

Third, "I can't help this patient." The issue of responsibility and helpfulness needs another look. The professional role is not something you put on overnight when you get your degree. You grow into it. As a clinical student, you are demonstrably more a clinician now than you were 2 years

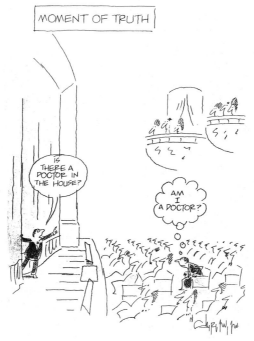

Drawing by Shirvanian; © 1985
The New Yorker Magazine, Inc.
Used by permission.

ago. Although still a learner, you are interacting with patients in a professional manner. The information you gather is important. Although the disease data you collect are only occasionally helpful, the personal data you collect will often contribute to the patient's well-being. If the patient has a specific request or complaint, you can discuss it with a unit nurse or resident. If the patient has a misunderstanding, you can clarify the problem or find somebody else to do so.

Finally, simply listening to patients in an empathic manner is usually therapeutic. Listening might not repair the damaged myocardium or lower the blood sugar level, but it will make the patient feel better. That is, after all, what clinical medicine is all about, although the primary goal of helping another person feel better often becomes confused, or at least seems remote, in a busy office or hospital. The patient is in a strange environment with a potentially serious or life-threatening illness and is caught in a system—an HMO, an office, or a hospital—that is not always flexible or responsive to human needs. If you are willing to take the time to listen, you will be surprised how therapeutic the encounter with you is for your patient, even though you are ostensibly "doing nothing." When the "moment of truth" comes (see the cartoon above), you will surprise yourself and be able to answer, "Yes, I am a doctor!"

S U M M A R Y : Science and Art in Interviewing

In this chapter we have stated one of the major themes of our approach to medical interviewing: the fact that conversation between clinician and patient is essential to both the science and the art of medicine. Because interviewing lies at the core of clinical science, we need to learn:

- Objectivity: Objectivity in clinician-patient interactions requires that we develop effective listening and responding skills.
  - o Letting the patient know you understand enhances objectivity.
  - o Jumping to premature interpretations compromises objectivity.
- Precision: This requires that the information we obtain be sufficiently detailed and unambiguous to use in diagnosis and treatment.
- Sensitivity: This requires that we use our interviewing skills to maximize our ability to identify "real" cases of illness.
- Specificity: This requires that we use our interviewing skills to maximize our ability to identify "real" cases of wellness.
- Reproducibility: In clinical situations, many factors contribute to the fact that different interviewers may obtain different stories from patients, but the use of good interviewing techniques will enhance reproducibility.

As shown in Figure 1–1, the science and the art of medicine are interdependent and synergistic. The fundamental skills enhance both.

Finally, a number of factors lead students who are just beginning to learn clinical interviewing to feel out-of-place, like fifth wheels. These factors, which may serve as barriers to learning and practicing new skills, include feeling as if you don't know enough, feeling reluctant to interact with patients who are tired and uncomfortable, and feeling awkward because you lack responsibility. In the next chapter, we explore the therapeutic core qualities, **respect, genuineness,** and **empathy,** which help overcome these barriers.

As we move on, basic skills used to obtain data from patients (objectivity, precision, reproducibility, sensitivity, and specificity) will enhance our ability to be empathic—that is, to *understand exactly* what patients are saying when they tell the stories of their illnesses.

References

1. Platt FW, McMath JC. Clinical hypocompetence: The interview. *Ann Intern Med* 1979; 91:898–902.
2. Rich EC, Crowson TW, Harris IB. The diagnostic value of the medical history. *Arch Intern Med* 1987; 147:1957–1960.
3. Kleinman A. *The Illness Narratives: Suffering, Healing, and the Human Condition.* New York, Basic Books, 1989.
4. Rogers C. *On Becoming a Person.* Boston, Houghton Mifflin, 1961.
5. Wright AD et al: Patterns of acquisition of interview skills by medical students. *Lancet* 1980; 2(8201):964–966.
6. Craig JL: Retention of interviewing skills learned by first year medical students: A longitudinal study. *Med Educ* 1992; 26:276–281.

Suggested Readings

Cassell EJ. *Talking With Patients. Volume 1, The Theory of Doctor-Patient Communication.* Cambridge, MA, MIT Press, 1985.

Cassell EJ. *Talking With Patients. Volume 2, Clinical Techniques.* Cambridge, MA, MIT Press, 1985.

Cohen-Cole SA. *The Medical Interview.* St. Louis, Mosby Year Book, 1991.

Feinstein AR. *Clinical Judgment.* Baltimore, Williams & Wilkins, 1967.

Smith RC, Hoppe RB. The patient's story: Integrating the patient- and physician-centered approaches to interviewing. *Ann Intern Med* 1991; 115:470–477.

CHAPTER 2

With Simple, Kindly Words

• • •

RESPECT, GENUINENESS, EMPATHY

He longed to soothe her, not with drugs, not with advice, but
with simple, kindly words . . .

Anton Chekhov, "A Doctor's Visit"

It is easy to agree that certain attitudes toward patients, such as genuineness and empathy, are praiseworthy. On first hearing this truism, you may think that these attitudes reflect the doctor's personality and value structure and are not immediately relevant to the medical history. You may not believe that these qualities are skills that can be learned and used. However, empathy and other qualities can, in fact, be understood as a certain set of behaviors. These behaviors can be practiced and learned.

In this chapter, we borrow some concepts from psychologists, particularly Carl Rogers and his followers, who first identified certain observable characteristics of the therapist that correlated with good therapeutic outcomes. They called these **therapeutic core qualities,** and the three most important were respect (or unconditional positive regard), genuineness (or congruence), and empathy. They found that the content of psychotherapeutic intervention, such as the specific intervention dictated by a theory, was less important to outcome than the process of the interactions. Subsequently, other investigators defined specific skills evident in that process. They showed that qualities such as empathy, for example, could be broken down into a set of skills in listening to and responding to a patient.[1]

These therapeutic core qualities are important links between the art and science of medicine. They improve the interviewer's history-taking ability and the accuracy of the data obtained, and they lead to better therapeutic relationships in ordinary practice. In the last chapter, we identified the goal of maximizing objectivity and precision in our communication with patients. In this chapter, we look at some generic concepts about how to do this before taking up the components of a medical history.

The following two examples serve to introduce these concepts. One is of a practicing physician interviewing a new patient in an office; the other is of a medical intern taking the history of a new patient in a clinic. In the first example, the patient is a 50-year-old woman who complains chiefly of abdominal pain that becomes worse when she gets upset:

Dr: What happens when you get upset? What do you feel like?

Pt: Oh, I just feel right nervous, the stomach pains, my arm . . . it pains, it seems like the strength is going out of my arm and hands.

Dr: How often do you get upset?

Pt: Quite frequently.

Dr: What's quite frequent?

Pt: Mostly every day it seems like I'm upset. I get something on my mind and that brings on the nauseated feeling.

Dr: So what's the usual sequence? You get upset first and then what happens? You get upset first or does the nausea come on first?

Pt: No. I get upset and then the nausea comes on.

Dr: What are you upset about?

Pt: Well, you know, things you want around the house there . . . it seems like things don't go right around the house. Like I get upset about that.

Dr: Tell me about when you started being upset.

Pt: Oh really, right after my mother passed, really, in April, I've been mostly upset.

Dr: What happened when your mother passed away? I understand it must have been a very upsetting event; was she very close to you?

Pt: Yes, I was really close to my mother, and it seems like after she passed, I don't know, something just left out of me, I don't know what it was, you know.

In the second example, the patient is a 40-year-old man who came for a checkup. The doctor is inquiring about his family history and found that the patient's father, who had divorced his mother, had died of a ruptured brain aneurysm:

Dr: You don't know anything more about that?

Pt: Well, my understanding is, the context of this is, that my mother was raised in the Catholic Church, and divorce was a terrible scandal in her mind and she tried to forget about it as quickly as she could. It's such a painful subject that there was never any discussion about who he was and so forth. And as a consequence all I've really heard are niblets, and one of the things I understand is that my father was an alcoholic or at least he had a problem with alcohol, but really caused my mother a lot of problems. So, I don't know if that would be a complicating factor in terms of an aneurysm or not.

Dr: Not that I know of. How about brothers and sisters?

Pt: I have one full natural brother and then four half brothers.

Dr: Medical problems in any of them that you know of?

Pt: No.

Dr: And you work as?

Pt: An editorial writer for the *Journal*.

Dr: And coming through your summer jobs, any unusual exposure to chemicals or mills or anything unusual that you did?

Pt: No, I worked in a bakery.

Dr: Asbestos?

All we have are transcripts of the tape recordings, so we can reconstruct neither the tone or quality of the language nor the nonverbal communication (e.g., head nods, eye contact, gestures). However, the physician in the first example (who, by the way, is a medical intern) appears to be connecting with the patient, acknowledging both the facts and the patient's feelings ("I understand it's a very upsetting event"). The physician in the second example does not appear to be on the same wavelength with the patient; the physician's agenda has little regard for the other person. The patient has told the physician that his father died of a cerebral hemorrhage, but he does not know anything else about it because his parents were divorced. The divorce, the "painful subject," and the history of alcoholism that pours out are ignored by the physician, who abruptly answers the patient's overt question and moves on ("Not that I know of. How about brothers and sisters?"). The second excerpt gives us a feeling that (at least in this interview) the interviewer's history-taking skills are not adequate.

As mentioned before, we can define three qualities that enhance communication between clinician and patient:

- **Respect:** The ability to accept the patient as he or she is and to avoid criticism.
- **Genuineness:** The ability to be one's self in a relationship despite one's professional role.
- **Empathy:** The ability to understand the patient's experience and feelings accurately, as well as to demonstrate that understanding to the patient.

Respect, genuineness, and empathy are qualities that we demonstrate in relationships with our patients by using specific communication techniques.

RESPECT

Respect means to value an individual's traits and beliefs despite one's own personal feelings about them and to see patients' feelings and behavior as a valid adaptation to their illness or life circumstances. Simply put, respect means being nonjudgmental. Some patients have irritating habits: smoking cigarettes, drinking too much, refusing to take medications, or even, at times, being antagonistic to their physicians or to clinical students. Other patients have beliefs about illness that try our patience: the man with severe emphysema might explain that his illness has nothing to do with his 100-pack-year smoking history but was caused by a cold he never got rid of in 1966. Another patient frustrates you with devastating migratory pains that refuse to go away, despite a normal examination and negative diagnostic tests. Some patients are obese or unable to keep themselves clean. Many have value systems different from yours or a healthy skepticism about the benefits of medical technology.

The skill in having respect is to separate your personal feelings about the patient's behavior or attitudes or beliefs from your basic concern—to help him or her get well. For example, the patient who believes that his emphysema is unrelated to smoking can still be guided to give a reliable account of his symptoms. Likewise, although the hostile patient makes you feel uncomfortable, you can still try to respect his or her reasons for being angry. Moreover, the emphysema patient's denial and the hostile patient's anger may actually be vital to their ability to tolerate their illnesses; such feelings should be accepted as part of the whole patient, not rejected as threats to the physician's ego. When patients act in ways that make you anxious or angry, they ordinarily have good reasons—based in their beliefs—for doing so, although they may be difficult for you to understand.

Respect involves valuing the patient as a person and as a historian. The following case example, taken from Platt and McMath,[2] demonstrates lack of respect in several ways:

> The interviewer failed to knock at the patient's door. He introduced himself in a hasty mumble so that the patient never had his name clearly in mind. He mispronounced the patient's name once and never used it again. The physician

conducted the interview while seated in a chair about 7 feet from the patient. There was no physical contact during the interview. On several occasions, the patient expressed her emotional distress. On each occasion, the interviewer ignored the emotional content of her statements.

Dr: Exactly where is this pain?

Pt: It's so hard for me to explain. I'm trying to do as well as I can. (Turning to husband:) Aren't I doing as well as I can?

Dr: Well, is the pain up high in your belly, or down low?

Pt: I kept getting weaker and weaker. I didn't want to come to the hospital. I was so frightened (weeping).

Dr: Did the pain come before the weakness or afterward?

The physical examination was brusque; the examiner never warned his patient when painful maneuvers (for example, firmly stroking the sole of the foot) were to be done. At the end of the examination, the physician failed to comment on his findings or his plans. He said in parting, "We'll do some tests and see if we can find out just what's the matter with you," and left the room before the patient had an opportunity to question him.

Notice how the physician seems to have his own agenda, ignoring the patient both as a person, by not acknowledging her emotional distress, and as a historian, by not helping to clarify the nature of the pain and weakness. This vignette illustrates a number of simple things you can do to demonstrate respect for your patient:

- You can introduce yourself clearly and communicate specifically why you are there. Since you are not the patient's friend, it would demonstrate lack of respect to use his or her first name during an initial interview without permission.
- You can inquire about and arrange for the patient's comfort before getting started and continue to consider his or her comfort during the course of your history and physical examination.
- You can conduct the interview while sitting at the patient's level, in a position where you can be easily seen and heard.
- You can warn the patient when you intend to do or say something unexpected or painful, particularly in the physical examination.
- You can respond to your patient in a way that indicates you have heard what he or she has said.

If the physician were demonstrating respect, the previous interview might have gone something like this:

Dr: Exactly where is the pain?

Pt: It's so hard for me to explain. I'm trying to do as well as I can. (Turning to husband:) Aren't I doing as well as I can?

Dr: I can see it's hard for you to explain and that you're trying hard. Perhaps you can show me where you are feeling it right now.

Pt: It's right about here (pointing) but what really frightened me was that I kept getting weaker and weaker and I didn't want to come to the hospital (weeping).

Dr: (Handing patient a box of tissues). Here, do you need one of these? Was it the weakness that frightened you?

Now the physician is focusing not only on the symptoms but also on the patient's feelings about the symptoms. In other words, the physician is communicating respect and, by so doing, is likely to acquire more accurate data more efficiently.

GENUINENESS

Genuineness means not pretending to be somebody other than who you are; it means being yourself, both as a person and as a professional. The first time you encounter this concept of genuineness as a problem in medicine may be in your role as a student. How do you introduce yourself? Should you introduce yourself as a clinical student or as a clinician? Do you allow a patient to address you as "doctor"? How do you respond when patients ask medical questions beyond your expertise or inquire about their own prognosis or care? Or when they say, "You look so young to be a doctor!" In all these cases, if you are to be genuine, you must acknowledge what you are: a student. You should introduce yourself as a student and, whenever appropriate, reaffirm to the patient your limited medical knowledge and limited responsibility (but not limited interest!) in the patient's care.

The term "student doctor" may represent a useful concept, both for you and for the patient. It acknowledges the patient's need—as well as your own—to perceive you in a professional, helping role, while it also genuinely describes what you are. If you are in medicine, "student doctor" more closely defines your role in the clinical encounter than does the more nondescript term "medical student." It also allows you to experience yourself in a more professional light and may facilitate your helping attitude toward the patient. On the other hand, you must make it clear to the patient that, "student doctor" or not, you are just learning.

Interns, residents, and practicing physicians all experience situations in which patients ask for opinions or require procedures beyond their capabilities. We may be required to call in consultants or refer patients to specialists. Genuineness requires you to be clear with the patient about what you do or do not know and can or cannot do, and to negotiate a plan for future care based on your capabilities. This aspect of genuineness is a component of being seen as trustworthy by your patients.

Being genuine also means being yourself in another way, that of expressing your feelings while staying within the bounds of a professional relationship. If a patient is in the hospital for a medical or surgical illness but has experienced a recent loss, such as the death of a spouse, it is desirable to respond to this fact with a statement such as, "I am sorry to hear that. How has it been going for you?" However, adding personal details (e.g., you too have lost a spouse or parent) may stress the limits of your comfort in a professional relationship. When patients say sad or comical things, it is appropriate to respond as a person and not just as a history-taker. Demonstrating your interest in the patient as a person is another way of being genuine.

There are situations, however, when respect and genuineness may seem contradictory. Everyone has bad days, and you may happen to be at a low ebb yourself during your evaluation of the patient. You may have been on call and up all night with a patient in the intensive care unit (ICU). You may be having problems in your personal life or be eagerly anticipating a weekend of skiing when you leave the hospital. At other times, you may be outraged about the patient's behavior, such as canceling or coming late to appointments. What is the role of genuineness in these situations? Should you hide your feelings, disguise your bad day, or express them to the patient? Although genuineness means not pretending, it does not mean that you must share all your feelings with the patient. You must distinguish your genuine professional self from the vicissitudes, experiences, or interests of your personal self. As you go through training, you gradually develop your professional self into a well-integrated instrument of healing. It is this professional self that serves as the standard for genuineness. For example, the patient who makes you angry by continually not showing up for appointments can be told that you, as a person, are angry about that, but, as a professional, you try to confine your anger to that aspect of the relationship. At the same time, you try to respect the patient by understanding his or her reasons for being late—chaotic lifestyle, three children younger than age 5, single parenting, need to take two buses to get to your office, and so forth.

This discussion leads to two caveats:

- It is rarely helpful to share your personal anger or disgust with the patient in the name of being honest. You may confront the patient with inconsistencies (to you) in his or her story or point out the patient's erratic behavior, if you believe it will help therapeutically; this is not the same as sharing your own negative feelings.

- Sometimes physicians are tempted to share their experiences and feelings as illustrations for the patient. This may range from statements like "I have young children too, and I know what you mean," to detailed personal anecdotes. Here again it is crucial to judge your personal revelations in the light of your professional judgment. Ordinarily, comments of rapport and connection are helpful. The type of car you own, the vagaries of parenting, or your opinions about a football team are not really self-revelations. On the other hand, it is rarely part of a genuine physician-patient interaction to describe intimate experiences or specific political or moral values.

Here is an example of a genuine response by a medical resident who is seeing a woman with asthma, peptic ulcer, and numerous psychosocial problems. The patient has just related a personal history of abuse during her childhood, and continues:

Pt: I can write a book. Well, you know, I'm not anymore, but I used to be atheist for awhile. God made me. I was a little girl, but I think about if you got children, you want the best for your children. If we are God's children, why did I go through what I went through? So that's why I feel the way I do.

Dr: I think about that all the time when I see people who are sick. They didn't bring it on themselves. It makes you wonder. No answer to that one.

EMPATHY

Empathy is a type of understanding. It is not an emotional state of feeling sympathetic or sorry for someone. Nor is it the same as the virtue of compassion. Although compassion may well be your motivation for developing empathy with patients, empathy is not compassion. In medical interviewing, being empathic means listening to the total communication—words, feelings, and gestures—and letting the patient know that you are really hearing what he or she is saying. The empathic physician is also the scientific physician because understanding is at the core of objectivity.

The skill in being empathic is in learning to talk to patients to maximize your ability to gather accurate data about their thoughts and feelings.

There are ways of responding to what patients say that will help you demonstrate to them that you understand. The data about specific symptoms that the patient gives you will be associated with feelings and beliefs. When you speak to patients, remember that you are speaking to a set of beliefs about the world.[3,4] The elderly gentleman who gives you a detailed description of his abdominal pain may at the same time feel frightened because he fears that the pain means stomach cancer because his father died of stomach cancer. His description will be filtered through his fears and his belief; unless you attend to the worry, the patient may not give an accurate account of what he is actually experiencing. One such patient may magnify the symptom to ensure a complete workup that will not miss cancer; another may minimize the symptom in the hope of being reassured that it is not cancer. If the interviewer acknowledges the fear, it is easier to get an accurate idea about what is really going on.

An empathic response can also be important in helping patients clarify their feelings. At times, the patient will not be in touch with his or her own feelings. By checking within yourself—how would you feel, for instance, upon finding blood in your stool?—you can formulate a response. Then, by checking back with the patient—by saying, for example, "That can be pretty frightening"—you as the interviewer can find out whether your assessment of what the patient might have felt is valid in that person's experience of illness.

LEVELS OF RESPONDING

It is useful to think of empathy as a feedback loop. You begin by listening carefully to what the patient is telling you, both cognitively and affectively. When you think you understand, you respond by telling the patient what you have heard. If you happen to be on the right wavelength, the patient will feel understood and be encouraged to reveal more of his or her thoughts and feelings. If you do not get it right, but yet have demonstrated your interest by checking back, the patient is likely to feel comfortable in correcting your impression, thus giving you an opportunity to reassess and respond again.

Your assessment of the strength of the feeling that the patient is experiencing will influence what you say to the patient—in other words, your level of response. If the patient believes that you are picking up on everything he or she says and are listening attentively with a nonjudgmental attitude, not only will accurate cognitive data emerge, but also feelings and beliefs. In formulating a response, it is important first to assess the nature and intensity of a feeling expressed. For example, is the patient upset? If so, is he or she slightly concerned or furious? Your assessment will include not only what the patient says but how it is said and how the patient looks when he or she says it.

In clinical interviewing you must learn a professional way of responding, which is different from the way you might respond in social interactions. In social situations, we often ignore or minimize feelings. For example, when people say, " 'How are you?" or "How do you feel today?," they do not ordinarily expect you to reveal how lousy you are actually feeling. In the clinical setting, however, you really do want to know the slings-and-arrows of how the person is feeling. You acknowledge the intensity of any feelings expressed and demonstrate that you understand and accept them. Consider these four categories or levels of responding: **ignoring, minimizing, interchangeable,** and **additive.**

Ignoring

You either do not hear what the patient has said or act as though you did not hear. You give no response to either the symptom content or feelings. For example:

Pt: Most days my arthritis is so bad the swelling and pain are just too much.
Dr: And have you ever had any operations?

---

and

Dr: Do emotional problems at work seem to make it worse?
Pt: I think it's . . .
Dr: Do coughing, sneezing, bending, straining at stool, any of those things make it worse?
Pt: I never associated it with those things.

Minimizing

You respond to the feelings and symptoms at less than the actual level expressed by the patient. For example:

Pt: I was in agony with the pain and terribly frightened.
Dr: Well, I'm sure it wasn't that bad.

---

and

Pt: Most days my arthritis is so bad the swelling and pain are just too much.
Dr: What you need is something to take your mind off it.

Interchangeable

You recognize the feelings and symptoms expressed by the patient and assess them accurately, and you feed back that awareness at the same level of intensity. For example:

Pt: Most days my arthritis is so bad the swelling and pain are just too much. I can't seem to do anything at all any more and nothing seems to help.
Dr: It sounds as though the pain and disability are really getting to you.

---

and

Pt: I was in agony with the pain and terribly frightened.

Dr: Severe pain can be pretty frightening. Was it the pain that scared you or the thought of what might be causing the pain?

The interchangeable response is a good response in medical history taking. It is usually a restatement in your own words of what the patient is trying to describe in order to communicate that you understand. When you give an interchangeable response, you are likely to find that it has a positive effect on the patient's ability to tell an accurate story. This kind of response is essential to being empathic.

In the following dialogue, the doctor responds to her patient's concerns even though she does not answer all the patient's questions right away:

Pt: But other than that I'm pretty good but it's my breasts I'm worried about. They started bleeding again, doctor. Why? I want you to take a look today. They're all bleeding in the inside. Is it anything to be concerned about?

Dr: Well maybe I can look and tell you.

Pt: Okay.

Dr: When did that start up again?

Pt: It seems like it will come and it will go, but now they're both all red and I noticed a whole lot of blood just drained out especially this right one, it really hurts down there. This side don't hurt me, but this side hurts me (touches her breasts). I don't know.

Dr: So you want me to take a look at your breasts (interchangeable response). Is that what's worrying you most today, your breasts? Is there anything else?

Pt: No.

Dr: Okay, come and let me take a look. (Patient and doctor move to examination table, and she begins checking patient.) Okay, I can see why you're so concerned; it looks pretty raw here. Okay, this is pretty much like it was before.

Pt: Yeah, but it really does hurt.

Dr: Yeah, I can see that it hurts (interchangeable response). This one is the worst, huh? Remember how well we were able to clear it up with medication the last time it got this bad?

Pt: Wonder what causes that. That's what worries me.

Dr: Yes, most women do worry about things that happen to their breasts (interchangeable response). But this is not serious, although it's very annoying and painful. When bleeding comes from inside the breast, it is serious. But this is from the skin. It's more like a skin allergy. The skin is real sensitive.

Pt: Oh, is that what it is? Okay.

How does one achieve an interchangeable response? Two concise ways are through mirrors and paraphrases. A mirror (or "reflection") simply feeds back to the patient exactly what is said:

Pt: I feel really terrible.
Dr: You feel really terrible?

A paraphrase conveys the same meaning as the patient's statement but uses different words.

Pt: I feel really terrible.
Dr: So you're really not feeling well, are you?

Additive

In an additive response, you recognize not only what the patient expresses openly but also what he or she may be unable to express. One common activity of physicians that involves using additive responses is that of reassurance. This involves making an educated guess regarding what the patient is likely to be worried about and dealing specifically with those worries. Here is an example of an additive response during a follow-up visit by a young man with headaches:

Dr: Well, how are you? Are you still having headaches?
Pt: Saturday I had a bad one. I wasn't able to sleep for five nights; my system is so pumped up I can't sleep. The pills did work. I took one a couple of hours before I went to bed and one just when I went to bed.
Dr: You mean the pills I gave you before you went to the hospital? Is it a red and yellow capsule?
Pt: Yeah. I took them two nights and last night was the first night I could sleep without them. I don't like to take a lotta stuff. I was having very strange effects from some of the medication.
Dr: Like what?
Pt: Well, you know everything else about me, I might as well tell you this. Those green pills made me . . . well, I can't describe the feeling it made me feel . . . very strange. They also depressed me, believe it or not, even

though you told me that they were antidepressants. I got depressed with them. For 2 days when I was taking them straight and in heavy doses, I found myself breaking into tears in situations . . . I don't even cry when I want to (laughs). It was very, very strange, so I stopped taking them.

Dr: So you're off them now?

Pt: Yeah, off everything now.

Dr: Okay. Can you tell me anything more about this strange feeling you had?

Pt: Ahhh . . . (patient hesitates)

Dr: Were you feeling like you were going to lose your mind? (additive response)

Pt: Yeah, I felt like I didn't have control over myself. I started to think I would get complications from the illness and how far behind it was making me get in my work because this is a very crucial time in my business. It really opened a lot of stuff for me. I never felt like this before.

The ability to achieve an additive response comes with the experience of listening carefully to patients' stories over time and learning patterns from them. Note that in the example above, the physician did not get it quite right. The additive response overshoots the patient's feeling, which was not so much "going to lose your mind" as it was "I didn't have control over myself." One of the benefits of an additive response is facilitating this kind of correcting, thereby improving accuracy.

For a patient with arthritis, an additive response might be:

Pt: Most days my arthritis is so bad the swelling and pain are just too much.

Dr: It sounds as though the pain is so bad that you think that things won't get much better.

If you have not gotten the sense of the statement quite right, the patient may respond:

Pt: Well, I do feel pretty bad, but I'm still hopeful.

Here is another example of an additive response, this time in an interview with a 50-year-old woman describing her history of depression:

Pt: You know, sometimes I scare myself.

Dr: You mean, you think about killing yourself?

Pt: Yeah, I do.

USING WORDS TO IDENTIFY SYMPTOMS AND FEELINGS

Symptom Words

To increase your skill in responding appropriately, it is necessary to pay attention to words, both your own and those of the patient. Premedical education and medical school can sterilize your vocabulary. You become immersed in the language of medicine, which, although very precise in describing some attributes, leaves little room for feelings or emotions. It is a language in which adjectives and adverbs carry little weight, and you are usually discouraged from using them in conversation. This socialization into the factual language of medicine can present real problems when you speak with patients. The world of the sick differs from the world of the well, but the difference does not include the sick learning the language of medicine. The most obvious problem you encounter with your medical vocabulary is that patients do not understand the words you use. When you say "hematemesis" rather than vomiting blood, or "paresthesias" rather than pins-and-needles sensations, your patient probably won't know what you are talking about.

Here is an example of a medical faculty member who was trying to ask a patient how much alcohol he drank:

Dr: Okay. Do you use ethanol a lot, little, weekends . . . ?
Pt: Tylenol?
Dr: Daily?
Pt: Ethanol? Alcohol?
Dr: Drinks?
Pt: You mean . . . alcoholic beverages? . . . I usually have a drink every night.
Dr: Okay.

The doctor was thinking "use ethanol" rather than "drink alcohol," and the choice of words created some confusion, which in this case was temporary. Fortunately, the patient acknowledged the misunderstanding. Many times patients do not let on that they have not understood your statement. This is a particular problem with yes/no questions and with explanations or instructions in which no response is sought from the patient.

Feeling Words, Qualifiers, and Quantifiers

Another important result of medical language and thought patterns is our often-impoverished ability to describe feelings, qualities, and emotions with any accuracy or precision. Empathy requires both accurate understanding and feeding back this understanding to the patient. This skill demands that

TABLE 2–1 DESCRIPTIVE WORDS FOR LEVELS OF FEELING

Intensity	Anger	Joy	Anxiety or Fear	Depression
Weak	Annoyed	Pleased	Uneasy	Sad
	Upset	Glad	Uncertain	Down
	Irritated	Happy	Apprehensive	Blue
Medium	Angry	Turned on	Worried	Gloomy
	Testy	Joyful	Troubled	Sorrowful
	Quarrelsome	Delighted	Afraid	Miserable
Strong	Infuriated	Marvelous	Tormented	Distraught
	Spiteful	Jubilant	Frantic	Overwhelmed
	Enraged	Ecstatic	Terrified	Devastated

we identify not only symptoms but also feelings, not only quantities but also qualities. Patients use words to quantify many symptoms: how much pain, how much blood, how much suffering, or how much vomiting. Although we are often more comfortable using numbers as quantities, patients frequently use analogies or comparisons to capture the intensity of their symptoms. For example, the patient who describes his pain as being as severe as a kidney stone is giving as precise a description as the patient who says that the pain is 8 on a scale of 1 to 10. Perhaps even more precise, as we may not know the patient's "10," but we do know that renal colic is one of the most severe pains a person can have.

Likewise, we must open up our windows to the world, and learn to use a broad vocabulary of feeling words. Table 2–1 presents examples of words that describe various emotions and their intensity. In giving an interchangeable response, you must "hit" not only the right feeling, but also the right intensity. The patient who says, "I am devastated by this pain" is not likely to believe you have really heard him or her if your response is, "So the pain upsets you a little?" On the other hand, when the patient mentions that "I feel a little crummy today," the physician is not sticking to his or her observations if the reply is "Sounds like you're feeling utterly hopeless." Once we accept the idea that medicine is about helping people to feel and function better, it is easy to understand how feelings reveal important data about the patient, which must be described as well as possible.

NONVERBAL COMMUNICATION

Nonverbal communication is the process of transmitting information without the use of words. It includes the way a person uses his or her body, such as facial expressions, eye contact, hand and arm gestures, posture, and various movements of the legs and feet. Nonverbal communication also includes paralinguistics—verbal qualities like tone, rhythm, pace, and vibrancy; speech errors; and pauses or silence. It is often through the nonverbal aspects of communication that we apprehend another's feelings. We recognize anger not so much by what a person says as by how it is said. Speech may slow down and get quiet in controlled anger, or the opposite may occur—with shouting and gestures such as pounding on a table. We can often tell when people lie unless they are good liars. They might look away, break eye contact, hesitate, or get "red in the face" (i.e., flush involuntarily). Common medical examples are the pressure of speech in the anxious or hypomanic person, or the flat voice tone of the very depressed. Patients who are ill often "sound" weak; we may gauge a person's state of health by how he or she sounds ("She's been through a lot of surgery, but she really sounds strong!").

Another component of nonverbal communication involves **kinesics**—that is, the use of personal space: how physically close we get to each other while talking to friends, business associates, lovers, patients. Other factors such as personal grooming, clothing, and odors (e.g., perspiration, alcohol, tobacco) also communicate information about the patient without words and can be helpful to you in understanding the situation. For example, if a patient who is normally careful about personal grooming comes in disheveled and unkempt, you are alerted to the possibility of a problem even before he or she begins to speak.

Even though the patient's nonverbal communication may be obvious to you, he or she is likely to be unaware of it. This does not mean that nonverbal messages are invalid; in fact, they may be more accurate than the verbal message, precisely because they are unintentional and uncensored. Although it is interesting to note various aspects of nonverbal communication, you may wonder what to do with your observations. Look for consistency; note nonverbal behaviors, and determine whether they are congruent with the patient's verbal message. When congruence exists, the communication is more or less straightforward. However, when there is a discrepancy, an effort must be made to ascertain which is the "real" message.

Here is an example of a patient who came in for a routine follow-up of abdominal pain and reported first that her husband, from whom she was separated, died recently of some sudden and unknown cause (he was 27 years old). David is the child they had together.

Pt: I want to tell you something before we start.

Dr: OK.

Pt: David's dad died. And now, it's like every week it's something new.

Dr: Oh my. (Note the genuine response.) What happened?

Pt: I don't know. He just went to sleep and never woke up.

Dr: My goodness, when did that happen?

Pt: Last Friday, right before the ninth.

Dr: Oh, I am so sorry to hear that. Ah, how is David doing?

The physician went on to explore how the patient and her son were reacting to this (usually) sad event, but the patient was discussing these issues with a bright smile on her face. Although she was separated from her husband, they had remained close because of David, and her cheeriness seemed inappropriate. What did the smile mean here? What kind of problem did this discrepancy suggest? Indeed, the physician seemed more upset about this news than the patient. It later came out that the patient was having great difficulty, particularly in communicating to her son appropriate ways to mourn and remember his father. Although the physician did not confront the patient early in the interview, he was alerted to a possible problem and later helped guide her toward a more appropriate response.

Often the nonverbal message is more accurate than the verbal statements. You may choose in some situations, especially early in the interview, simply to note a discrepancy and use it to help you understand the patient. Or you might use the nonverbal communication to modify your own nonverbal behavior, your conversation, or both. For example, if the patient seems tense, as evidenced by facial flushing or fidgeting, you may modify your voice tone and the way you are sitting in response to the patient's discomfort by speaking in a more soothing way and leaning forward to demonstrate your interest.

At the same time that you are observing the patient's nonverbal behavior, the patient is, perhaps unconsciously, observing your nonverbal behavior as well. As a result, your job is twofold: You should be aware of your own nonverbal behavior, as well as the patient's. For example, if you seem uninterested, as evidenced by never looking at the patient or by looking at your watch, he or she may be unable to provide the details you need. Likewise, if you stand by the door as opposed to sitting by the bed, patients may assume you are in a hurry and, respectful of your time, leave out critical data they decide are unimportant. Attention to your own nonverbal behavior requires a high level of self-awareness and discipline. It is particularly important to be conscious of how you respond to distractions during the interview, such as an emergency across the hall. You need to demonstrate your focus on the patient by maintaining eye contact, an attentive posture, and a seeming lack of awareness that all hell is breaking loose somewhere else.

Gestures

Although specific gestures have been the subject of study and suggested interpretations, their meanings must always be judged in context. When the gesture or facial expression appears to imply something different than the words, an effort must be made to ascertain which—the gesture or the words—is delivering the real message. Interpretation is no problem when a gesture "confirms" the patient's statements or the doctor's hypothesis based on them. Consider this example in which a patient is suffering from headaches. The physician learns that the patient has been under much stress recently.

Dr: So you have a lot of things on your mind.

Pt: Yes. About them, about some of the members of my family, and, um, mostly it's money worries, mainly money. (Patient puts her hand on the part of her head that has been painful.)

Dr: It's funny, when you say "money worries," you know where you point to?

Pt: Huh?

Dr: You point right where it's hurting.

Pt: Yeah, ah hah. . . . That's mostly it, you know.

In this situation, pointing out the relationship between financial stress (verbal) and tension headaches (nonverbal, pointing to head) might well be effective both in demonstrating your empathic understanding and in making explicit a connection the patient may already experience implicitly.

Table 2–2 presents a list of common gestures and some of their suggested interpretations. Two of these deserve comment. The helplessness or

TABLE 2–2 GESTURES AND POSSIBLE INTERPRETATIONS

Gesture	Possible Interpretation
"Steepling" of hands involves joining them with fingers extended and fingertips touching, like a church steeple	Confidence or assurance of what is being said
Slight raising of the hand or index finger, pulling at an earlobe, or raising the index finger to the lips	A desire to interrupt the speaker
Helplessness or hopelessness gesture (see text)	Feeling of hopelessness; a request for help is futile
Respiratory avoidance response (see text)	Rejection of or disagreement with what is being said
Raising a finger to the lips	An attempt to suppress a comment
Crossed arms (note the manner in which the arms are crossed and muscular tension, especially in the hands)	A defensive gesture indicating disagreement, a sign of insecurity, or simply a comfortable position
Increased muscle tension, "white knuckle syndrome"	Fear or tension
Crossed legs	An attempt to shut out or protect against what is going on in the interview, or simply a position of comfort
Uncrossed legs, shifting forward in the chair	Receptivity to what is going on in the interview

hopelessness gesture is typically biphasic. Both hands are raised briskly to face level, with elbows fixed, palms facing each other; they are rotated slightly outward, fingers spread, and thumb and fingers slightly flexed as though preparing to grasp. This position is held briefly, and then the hands fall limply down to the lap. This gesture suggests that the patient feels helpless about the problem or situation. The first part may represent reaching out for assistance, while the second part (hypotonia and withdrawal) emphasizes the futility of receiving any help.

The respiratory avoidance response includes frequent clearing of the throat when no phlegm or mucus is present. A variation of this is the nose rub, which involves a light rub of the nose with the dorsal aspect of the index finger. These gestures indicate rejection or disagreement with statements being made. For example: "How are things at home?" The patient answers "Fine," clears his throat, and lightly rubs his nose. He may actually be saying, "Things aren't really going very well at home."

Paralanguage

When you hear a patient's speech, you hear pauses, tone, and modulation, in addition to words. Likewise, the patient hears the pitch and rhythm of your converstation. Table 2–3 lists the elements of **paralanguage**. Paralinguistic cues can contribute significantly to your understanding of the patient and to the patient's perception of you as a helping person.

Let us deal briefly with just one aspect of paralanguage: pauses. The patient pauses a moment before answering your question, or before making her next statement. Why does she pause? The functions of pausing include:

- Absolute recall time
- Language formation time
- Censorship of material
- Creating an effect (timing)
- Preparing to lie

TABLE 2–3   COMPONENTS OF PARALANGUAGE

Component	Examples
Speech rate	Slow, fast, deliberate
Pauses	Long, short, inappropriate
Pause/speech ratio	Mechanical, halting, flowing speech
Tone or voice quality	Whiny, flat, nasal, bright, breathy
Pitch	High, medium, low
Volume	Loud, soft, wide variations
Articulation	Clear, precise, slurred

Adapted from Cassell with permission.[4]

People rarely need to pause before recalling a place, age, or date fixed in time. For example, a person readily remembers the age at which a parent died, but might have to think a moment before remembering a living parent's current age. It is easy to answer a "yes/no" question without pausing, even if giving the incorrect answer: "Do you drink alcohol?" Yes. No. This has little meaning. Alternatively: "How much alcohol do you usually drink in a day?" or "Tell me about your use of alcohol." These questions demand some thought and integration. Listen carefully. How much of a pause occurs before the answer? How much stumbling or backtracking?

In general, it is helpful to listen to the number, quality, and placement of pauses. Frequent long pauses associated with low amplitude and a "dead" tone suggest depression. Frequent pauses over factual answers throughout the history suggest dementia or organic brain dysfunction. Pauses over answers in selected areas may indicate sensitive topics, with time required for censorship of material. We return to this aspect of medical interviewing later in this book, in the sections on truth telling and difficult interviews.

CHALLENGES TO UNDERSTANDING EXACTLY

Some history-taking situations present unavoidable technical difficulties. These include, for example, language barriers, the patient's state of consciousness (comatose, delirious, psychotic, or demented), and the patient's educational level or language skills. Two examples follow. In the first, an interview with an Iranian woman was proceeding well until the physician asked the patient if she had any "allergies," clearly a difficult word to translate:

Dr: And do you have cough? (Demonstrates)
Pt: No, no cough.
Dr: Fever? Hot? (Touches forehead)
Pt: Yes, yes, I feel hot.
Dr: Uh, allergy to medicine? Pill give you rash? Reaction? (Points all over skin, scratching to get at idea of itchy rash)
Pt: (Looking confused) I don't know.
Dr: Excuse me, I'll get your brother to help us speak.

In the following encounter with an elderly, demented patient, the patient simply cannot remember his recent symptoms; rather, he is only aware of how he feels at present:

Dr: Do you know who I am?
Pt: Well, I don't know, no.

Dr: I'm Dr. Smith.

Pt: Oh.

Dr: I'm glad to see you today. How have you been feeling?

Pt: Oh, I don't know, just all poured out.

Dr: Weak, are you weak?

Pt: I imagine to a certain extent, but it seems just that nothing just seems to be right.

Dr: (Taking pulse) Your pulse feels good today.

Pt: I'm glad there's something good about me.

Dr: Do you feel there's not much good about you?

Pt: Oh well, I guess I'm just average.

Dr: How's your heart been treating you?

Pt: Oh, it never did bother me.

Dr: How are you sleeping at night?

Pt: No trouble at all.

Dr: How's your appetite?

Pt: Always with me.

In such situations, we ordinarily dismiss the possibility of a useful interview with the patient and seek information elsewhere. In our examples, the physician obtained an interpreter for the Iranian woman and spoke with the demented patient's wife. In fact, she stated that his appetite was poor, he was having a lot of trouble sleeping, and he was frequently short of breath. You should be aware, however, that language barriers are sometimes subtle: the patient might miss just a few crucial words. Likewise, dementia may be mild and variable. You need to listen carefully for inappropriate responses or evidence of confusion. It is useful early in the interview to detect technical problems that will lead to faulty data collection. Only then are you ready to proceed with eliciting the chief complaint and history of the present illness.

S U M M A R Y : Core Therapeutic Skills

In this chapter we have presented three fundamental skills of clinician-patient interactions:

- Respect
- Genuineness
- Empathy

We have described what each skill means in the medical interview, and behavioral techniques to enhance the skill.

Empathy means understanding exactly what the patient is saying and letting the patient know that you understand. To enhance empathy in the clinical encounter:

- Strive for interchangeable responses.
- Develop and use a good vocabulary of descriptive words.
- Pay attention to nonverbal communication, especially paralinguistics.

Armed with an understanding of these fundamental skills, you are now ready to begin the interview, as we move on to Chapter 3.

References

1. Ivey AE, Authier J. *Microcounselling*. Springfield, IL, Charles C Thomas, 1978.
2. Platt FW, McMath JC. Clinical hypocompetence: The interview. *Ann Intern Med* 1979; 91:898–902.
3. Cassell EJ. *The Healer's Art*. Philadelphia, JB Lippincott, 1976.
4. Cassell EJ. *Talking With Patients. Volume 1, The Theory of Doctor–Patient Communication*. Cambridge, MA, MIT Press, 1985.

Suggested Readings

Cassell EJ. *Talking With Patients. Volume 2, Clinical Techniques*. Cambridge, MA, MIT Press, 1985.

Coulehan JL. Being a physician. In: Mengel MB, Holleman W (Eds.). *Fundamentals of Clinical Practice. A Textbook on the Patient, Doctor, and Society*. New York, Plenum Medical Book Company, 1997, pp. 73–101.

Lavasseur J, Vance DR. Doctors, nurses, and empathy. In: Spiro H, Curnen MGM, Peschel E, St. James D (Eds.). *Empathy and the Practice of Medicine*. New Haven, CT, Yale University Press, 1993, pp. 76–84.

More ES. "Empathy" enters the practice of medicine. In: More ES, Milligan MA (Eds.). *The Empathic Practitioner. Empathy, Gender, and Medicine*. New Brunswick, NJ, Rutgers University Press, 1994, pp. 19–39.

Platt FW, Keller VF. Empathic communication: A teachable and learnable skill. *J Gen Intern Med* 1994; 9:222–226.

Spiro H. What is empathy and can it be taught? *Ann Intern Med* 1992; 116:843–846.

CHAPTER 3

Why Should You Come to Consult Me?

• • •

THE CHIEF COMPLAINT AND PRESENT ILLNESS

"Never mind," said Holmes, laughing; "it is my business to know things. Perhaps I have trained myself to see what others overlook. If not, why should you come to consult me?"

Arthur Conan Doyle, "A Case of Identity"

from *The Adventures of Sherlock Holmes*

In the next four chapters we discuss the traditional parts of a complete medical history—that is, the chief complaint, present illness, other active problems, past medical history, family history, social history or patient profile, and review of systems. In each section we introduce, describe, and illustrate skills or techniques useful for that part of the interview—skills particularly appropriate to the content or medical objective (e.g., the review of systems requires a different approach than the history of the present illness). This division of the interview is for simplicity of illustration only and does not imply that open-ended questions or interchangeable responses, for example, are useful only in the "present illness" section. Remember, too, that one does not necessarily proceed in this order or, for that matter, in one sitting.

Sometimes the family history is obtained in the opening moments of the encounter ("My mother had breast cancer, so I thought I'd better come in for a check-up"); or the patient profile evolves over several encounters with the patient.

This chapter deals with (1) the setting, (2) getting started, (3) the chief complaint, and (4) the present illness.

THE SETTING

In the past clinicians usually first learned their interviewing skills with hospitalized patients. Although the emphasis is now on ambulatory care, students still frequently begin their experience in the hospital setting. The hospital is an unnatural habitat; as a result, the patient, who is "diseased," may not feel at ease. Patients may be similarly uncomfortable, although perhaps less so, in the HMO or physician's office. When you see a patient for the first time, his or her blood pressure and pulse are often elevated, the face flushed, the handshake cool and damp, and the gestures clearly nervous. These characteristic signs indicate the autonomic response to the stress of illness, seeking help, meeting a new doctor, and the possibly unknown procedures and outcome. If you appear hurried, indifferent, or unsympathetic, the patient is likely to feel even more uncomfortable; this discomfort creates a barrier to effective communication.

GETTING STARTED

The beginning of the interview sets the atmosphere for the rest of your history and physical examination. Quickly show your respect with a friendly greeting and begin by establishing a sense of privacy for the interview. For example, if there is another patient sharing the hospital room, draw the curtain around the bed. Even though this obviously does not provide a soundproof barrier, it provides the patient with a psychologic sense of privacy. If the patient can walk comfortably, it may be better to interview him or her in a convenient lounge or waiting area, if this would be more private. If the patient has visitors, you might suggest that they wait outside or, if possible, that you will return later to see the patient. Before beginning the history, check to see that the patient is as comfortable as possible. Try to seat yourself in a way that will facilitate communication. People have spheres of "personal space": Get close enough for a person-to-person interaction, but do not intrude on the patient's intimate space.

In a small hospital room it may be difficult to place yourself comfortably so that you strike a balance between being halfway across the room and sitting on top of the patient. If necessary, move your chair. Try to sit at the same level as the patient; this helps establish good eye contact during the interview. Often it is most comfortable to sit at an angle to the person, rather than facing him or her directly: This allows you to maintain good eye contact, but also provides natural opportunities to look away at times. Good eye contact does not mean staring fixedly, which will only make the patient feel uncomfortable; there are always natural breaks in eye contact. You can also use your body to demonstrate interest: leaning slightly toward the patient rather than lounging back in your chair.

Consider these guidelines:

- **Introduce yourself and explain your role.** Although local policies differ, if you are a student, we strongly suggest you introduce yourself as such. Besides being genuine and not using a professional facade, you will also be defining your limited **contract** with the patient. The patient expects to describe a complaint and then to have the doctor treat it. If you are a student who does not have responsibility to care for the patient, the contract is different. When the patient asks your opinion about his or her diagnosis or treatment, asks for pain medication, or requests anything outside your capacity to respond, you can comfortably remind the patient of the boundaries of your contract. You can tell the patient that you will convey the question to the resident or nursing staff, or suggest that the patient do so.

- **Don't begin by saying, "I've been asked (or sent) to take a history and do a physical."** Such a statement is likely to make the patient feel that you have no real interest in him or her and may set the interview off on the wrong track. A better start would be to say, "I'd like to talk to you today in order to get some information about why you're in the hospital, and then to examine you. Will that be all right?" As part of this introduction, you obtain permission (the contract) to do the history and examination; by so doing, you demonstrate respect for the person.

- **Taking notes is essential** because you will be writing up the information you obtain. As you begin, inform the patient of your need to take notes and the reason for it; this will also let the patient know what will happen to the information you are obtaining. However, try not to let your note taking control the interview. If you attempt to record the conversation verbatim—with the exception of the chief complaint—the patient is likely to feel that he or she is being interrogated rather than being interviewed. Moreover, the process of taking so many notes will interfere with the flow of the conversation. Eye contact will be severely limited if you are mainly concerned with note taking, and you are likely to miss the nonverbal communication, thereby interfering with rapport and missing useful data about the person. While you are making notes, look up frequently; this will demonstrate your interest. You will find with more experience that only an occasional word or phrase needs to be written down to help you remember, synthesize, and later reconstruct the story in complete written form.

THE CHIEF COMPLAINT

The **chief complaint** in a standard medical history is the main reason why the patient sought medical help. **It is usually recorded verbatim in the patient's own words.** The chief complaint is often elicited by such questions as:

- How can I help you today? (If you have responsibility for the patient.)
- Can you tell me about your trouble?
- What symptoms made you decide to see a doctor/come to the emergency room?
- Can you tell me about your problem?
- Tell me about the main thing you feel is wrong.
- What brought you to the hospital? (Although this question may be subject to concrete answers like, "A taxi.")
- Tell me why you had to come to the emergency room today.

Consider this example of how one medical resident began an interview with a new patient in an outpatient clinic:

Dr: I guess the best place to start is to ask you what brings you here today.

Pt: Well, I haven't had a physical really for 6 years now, since my daughter was born.

Dr: I am going to be writing some things down on paper here, okay? Is there any particular reason why you chose now to come in?

Pt: I figured I kept putting it off and putting it off. I'd make appointments and put them off. There is no particular reason. I just felt as though it was time, I suppose.

Dr: Nothing is bothering you at this point?

Pt: No, it's just that I am overweight, that's all. I go up and down, up and down.

Dr: So that was your major concern, the weight problem?

Pt: Yeah.

Dr: Can you tell me about that?

The chief complaint, stated verbatim, is: "It's just that I am overweight." It took a little digging to clarify that; the physician was appropriately not satisfied with "There is no particular reason."

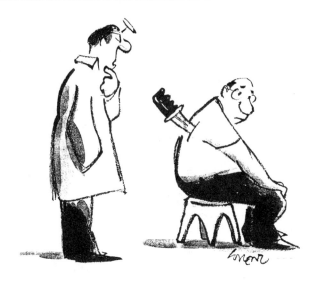

*"It's got to come out, of course, but that doesn't address
the deeper problem."*

Drawing by Lorenz; © 1988
The New Yorker Magazine, Inc.
Used by permission.

Sometimes an opening question leads to a clear-cut chief complaint, as in this example:

Dr: What can I do for you?

Pt: Um, the reason why I'm here is, since the latter part of July up to now, my bowels wouldn't move and I'd have to, in like 4 and 5 days, I'd have to take either milk of magnesia or a bulk laxative, and I just thought it was maybe something that I was eating, and this still continues until now, and it's the reason why I'm here to see you.

In other cases, the same opening question might lead to a much more complex and rambling answer:

Dr: Now what can I do for you, Mrs. P?

Pt: Well, first of all, I'm here mainly because I've been experiencing that tired, worn-out feeling most of the time. I can go to bed, say 9:00 in the evening, and get up at 8:00 or even later and I still feel very tired. And, I don't know . . I've still been experiencing hot flashes and sometimes now . . I don't experience them as often as I used to, but I still do, especially towards the evening or at night, and it awakens me when I do experience something like that. Maybe that's part of the reason why I felt so tired, I don't know. Anyways, now in the evening when I experience this kind of hot feeling, I just get that craving— I want to eat, you know, or sometimes it works just the opposite where I feel kind of nervous, I get that nervous feeling, and now last week I had headaches just about every day on arising; I had a little runny nose, so maybe, I don't know, maybe I could attribute that to a cold, but I'm just mentioning those things to you. And, sometimes you know my head just feels as though . . . it feels stuffed . . . when you have a head cold; that's just the way it has felt many times. And I had a hysterectomy, let's see, about 1986 or '87 and since then I just have had no sexual desire or anything. I mean, as far as I'm concerned that doesn't mean a whole lot. I know it upsets my husband a bit.

What is the chief complaint? Ostensibly, it is her first statement, "mainly because (of) that tired, worn-out feeling . . ," but, in context, the situation is less clear. What is really bothering her most? Why did she come here today, as opposed to last month or next week? This patient rambles on and on, presenting a challenge to the interviewer that we will discuss near the end of this chapter (p. 60). The physician permits this lengthy response, and, in so doing, acquires a wealth of useful information about the patient's symptoms and concerns. The physician will later establish more structure for the patient to clarify her complaints. In contrast to this example, Beckman and Frankel[1] found that in only 23 percent of office visits did medical residents allow the patient to complete his or her opening statement. Rather, in most cases they interrupted and steered the discussion toward a specific topic, thereby diminishing the chance of getting to the patient's real chief complaint.

However, it is not just the discursive patient who presents problems in identifying the chief complaint; often, the actual reason why the person comes to see the physician lies embedded somewhere else, far from the patient's initial statement (see cartoon on p. 46). Here is an example of a patient who presents with chest pain that he has had for some time:

Dr: I'm glad you came in today. Tell me why you came in.

Pt: Okay. I been having some problems with my chest; you know it's, it's like pressure and plus I have a knot under my arm, under my armpit.

Dr: Okay. You have pressure.

Pt: Yeah, I have pressure, and I don't know if it's because I smoke a lot of cigarettes, or I don't know what it is.

Dr: Um hum.

Pt: All I know is it's pressure across my chest. It's not what you call a pain or anything—it hurts; it's pressure all across here.

Dr: Um hum.

Pt: And, then, I have this knot under my, under my armpit.

Dr: Okay.

Pt: About the size of a half dollar.

Dr: Okay, let's talk about the chest pain first; when would you say it started?

Pt: Um, I'd say about a month ago; maybe it might have been longer but I didn't pay it any attention.

Dr: Um hum.

Pt: You know but I can't jog because if I just start jogging, it bothers me in my chest.

Dr: What made you decide to get it checked?

Pt: Well, two things actually, I want to get back in shape and I got a note from the Health Department that this test came back positive. See I'm a barber and they test for tuberculosis.

By asking "What made you decide to get it checked?" this physician not only has the answer to why the patient came in now, but also an important new piece of data—namely the positive tuberculin test result. We also learn that the patient may believe there is a relationship between his symptoms and the positive tuberculin test result. He really came to the doctor because of the test result, perhaps simply to fulfill a legal requirement for his license, and perhaps, in addition, because the test result made him reinterpret his chest problems as being more serious than he thought they were. In any case, if the work-up for tuberculosis is negative, the physician knows that the patient will need reassurance that the cause of his trouble does not lie in the positive tuberculin test result.

When you consider why a person might come for medical help at a certain time, it is not enough simply to elicit the symptoms. The symptoms, as in the previous example, may have been present for some time. Although the answer to a question like "How can I help you?" frequently contains the core of the patient's problem, sometimes it does not. The **ostensible reason for coming**, as initially stated by the patient in the chief complaint, may not be the same as the **actual reason for coming**.[2] This is most often true with:

- People who have chronic diseases
- People with vague, chronic, and/or recurring symptoms
- People who say they just want a checkup

Alvan Feinstein[3] used the term **iatrotropic stimulus** (iatrotropic = toward the physician) to indicate why the patient decided to seek care today rather than yesterday, tomorrow, or last year. If you can answer the question "Why now?" you have probably uncovered the iatrotropic stimulus or the actual reason for coming. Despite the fact that the person has an "acceptable" symptom or disease (congestive heart failure or shortness of breath), it may not satisfactorily explain why the patient is here today, and what he or she expects.

Why do patients seek care at a particular time?

- First, the symptoms of the illness may increase to the point that they become unbearable and the person simply realizes he or she needs medical help. We usually assume this reason, and it is often quite true in acutely ill patients.

- Second, anxiety about the meaning of the symptoms may, for one reason or another, reach the point where the person seeks medical help, even though he or she may have been sick for quite a while, or may even have had a decrease in symptoms. Perhaps a TV news story about a certain disease or the recent diagnosis of a brain tumor in a friend increases anxiety about an otherwise trivial symptom, such as a headache.

- Third, the symptom in the chief complaint is sometimes a **"ticket of admission"** to the physician's office or emergency room; the actual problem may be an entirely different symptom that the patient is at first afraid to mention, or it may be some life stress or crisis.

Finally, if you really listen, the iatrotropic stimulus will come out during the interview. Sometimes it arrives only at the last moment, when you are about to walk out of the room and the patient says, "Oh, by the way, Doc, I'm sure this has nothing to do with it, but . . ."[4] We will discuss the "Oh, by the way" or "doorknob" phenomenon later, in Chapter 9. However, basic respect, empathy, and open-ended questioning early in the interview go a long way toward minimizing or avoiding that phenomenon. The earlier in the interview you ascertain the patient's reason for coming, the more efficient you will be, wasting less time digging for data. For example, the patient with the rambling "chief complaint" whom we met earlier in this chapter actually provides all of her concerns within the opening 2 minutes of the interview. The clinician can take notes and come back to each in turn, prioritizing for maximum efficiency. We will return to this technique in Chapter 9, when we discuss primary care interviewing.

THE PRESENT ILLNESS

The **present illness** is a thorough elaboration of the chief complaint and other current symptoms starting from the time the patient last felt well until the present. The best strategy for this part of the interview is often, first, to let the patient talk, then to use a variety of nondirective and directive questions to clarify and embellish. Generally you move from open-ended questions to more specific "Wh" questions (who, what, when, where, why, and how), laundry list questions (menus), or closed-ended questions, as appropriate, to achieve precision in symptom description.

Open-Ended Questions

Some examples are:

- Can you tell me more about that?
- Did you notice anything else?
- What was the pain like for you?

Another version of these open-ended questions is to restate them as gentle commands, requesting the patient to elaborate:

- Tell me more about that.
- Tell me what else you noticed.
- Tell me what the pain was like.

Nondirective or open-ended questions are always a good way to start, allowing the patient freedom to talk and the examiner time to sit back and "size up" the patient. They are especially good for eliciting the less structured data of the present illness and the psychosocial aspects of the patient's problem. These questions allow the patient, who, after all, is the one who knows the story, to choose the most important symptoms and to point the way. The most nondirective of all statements are **minimal facilitators**—queries like:

- "Yes?"
- "Uh huh?"
- "And?"
- "And what else?"

Nonverbal cues, such as nodding your head in agreement or smiling, also may serve as minimal encouragement for the patient to continue talking.

Wh Questions

Nondirective questioning usually just sketches the picture, without giving precise detail. Patients only rarely spontaneously volunteer all the needed details; a rambling, vague patient may take too much time and still not provide the information you need, while a shy, reticent patient may say little or nothing. So in a medical interview you move from the general to the more directive, but still open-ended, **Wh questions**. These describe the attributes of the patient's symptoms and specify the story.

WHERE	Exactly where is it on your body? *or* Show me where it is.
WHAT	What does it feel like? *or* Tell me what it feels like.
WHEN	When did it start? Does it come and go, or does it stay? When does it occur (episodic, inception and duration, fluctuation, and frequency)?
HOW	How is it altered by season, by time of day, by sleep, by

food, by exertion, and so forth? Describe how your daily activities affect it.

WHY — Why do you think it occurs? Why do you think you have this problem?

WHO — Who is affected by it? (consequences to patient and other people)

Directive and Closed-Ended Questions

Patient disclosure of relevant clinical information is most strongly correlated with open-ended questions, but other types of questions are usually also necessary to develop the patient narrative. **Laundry list questions,** or **menus,** are sometimes useful when a patient cannot find words to express a certain characteristic. For example, "How would you describe this pain—sharp, dull, burning, or tight?" "Would you say it lasted a few seconds, a minute, 10 minutes?" Such questions obviously exclude other descriptive words and should be used only when a nondirective approach ("Can you describe the pain?") and Wh questions ("What is the pain like?") have both failed.

Directive, or **closed-ended, questions** provide detail; they are good for emergency situations ("What's your name?" "How old are you?" "Are you allergic to any drugs?"), for reticent patients, and for structured data, such as the past history and the review of systems. They are also useful as focused questioning when you have already generated hypotheses in the interview and are trying to build a case for one particular diagnosis. However, a "high control" interview in which the interviewer asks one directive question after another will produce false or incomplete evidence, not to mention a discontented patient. Some other examples of closed-ended questions are:

- Are your parents still living?
- Did you actually pass out?
- Have you ever been anemic?
- Does this pain occur when you take a deep breath?
- Is there any trouble with your vision?

One does not ask yes/no questions in situations in which information may be sensitive, because a lie will close off all access to that information. For example, it is not useful to say, "Do you drink alcohol?" if one suspects alcohol may be a problem; try, "How much alcohol do you usually drink in a day?"

Finally, there are at least two types of questions to avoid.

- **Avoid leading questions,** which encourage certain responses from the patient to fit the interviewer's own hypothesis, such as "You're feeling better now, aren't you?" or "That pain wasn't on the left side of your chest, was it?" This type of query suggests to the patient what you want (or don't want) to hear.

- Likewise, **avoid multiple questions**, such as: "Do you have any trouble sleeping and how about coughing?" Sometimes these slip out, because your mind is working too quickly and dragging your tongue along with it. Slow down; wait. Table 3–1 summarizes the various types of queries employed in taking the medical history.

Symptom Description

Throughout the history of the present illness, it is important to describe the patient's symptoms as carefully as possible without jumping to conclusions. For example, "I'm short of breath" does not necessarily indicate dyspnea on exertion or orthopnea; it could be fatigue, weakness, or angina. It is also important to avoid jumping to conclusions about the meanings of words. Many words popularly used to describe symptoms mean different things to different people. Some examples are diarrhea, constipation, tired, dizzy, my side, sick, weak, high blood, low blood, insomnia, gas, and heartburn. The novice has a tendency to establish quantitative aspects of symptoms ("How many times a day?") before establishing the qualitative aspects. The expert interviewer attempts to establish what he or she is dealing with ("Are the stools soft or watery?") before measuring it. You want first to establish the pattern, or *gestalt*; then you should fill in the quantitative data. Table 3–2 presents examples of patient statements, followed by either quantitative (prematurely specific) or qualitative follow-up questions.

It is also important not to get caught up in the "New Brunswick syndrome" when taking the patient's history. A friend of ours was living in Canada and his mother from New Jersey was visiting. They were invited to a party and our friend noted that his mother was carrying on a long, animated discussion with a woman with whom he thought she had nothing in common. Afterward, he asked his mother what they were talking about. She said, "Well, we were sharing a lot of memories of our childhoods in New Brunswick." They had carried on a long, gratifying conversation despite the

TABLE 3–1 TYPES OF QUESTIONS IN THE MEDICAL INTERVIEW

Start with	Open-ended questions (general) Open-ended questions (topical) Minimal facilitators
Proceed to	Wh questions Laundry lists of menus Closed-ended questions "Yes/no" questions
Avoid	Leading questions Complex/multiple questions

TABLE 3–2 REPORTED SYMPTOMS: EXAMPLES OF QUANTITATIVE AND QUALITATIVE CLINICIAN QUESTIONS

Complaint	Quantitative Questions	Qualitative Questions
I've been having chest pain.	How long have you had it? How often does it come?	What does it feel like? Where exactly is it located?
My side hurts.	How long have you had it?	Show me where.
I have diarrhea.	How many times a day?	What do you mean by diarrhea?
I vomited blood.	How much?	What did it look like?
I can't walk as far as I used to without getting tired.	How far can you walk?	What do you mean by "tired?"

fact that one was talking about New Brunswick, New Jersey, and the other was referring to the Canadian province of New Brunswick. The same words mean different things to different people. This does not present much of a problem at a cocktail party, but it can be deadly in the clinical interview.

The symptom called "dizziness" presents a prime example. A patient comes in and says, "My main problem is dizziness. It just came on me about a month ago, and it's been getting worse now. I'm so dizzy I can hardly stand up sometimes. What's wrong with me, Doc?" The first thing wrong is the word "dizziness." There are at least four symptoms commonly labeled with this word:

- Vertigo, a definite sense of rotation or environmental motion
- Presyncope, the sensation that loss of consciousness is about to happen
- Disequilibrium, the sensation that balance, especially during walking, is impaired
- Lightheadedness, a vague head sensation that is not vertigo and not presyncope

Some people also idiosyncratically label weakness, fatigue, or anxiety as dizziness.

The following exchange, adapted from Reilly,[5] shows an example of a physician trying to find out precisely what a patient means by dizziness:

Dr: Can you describe what you mean with words other than dizzy?

Pt: I feel out of balance. I feel like I might fall down even. I haven't yet, but I get awful woozy when I walk.

Dr: Is it mainly when you walk that you have trouble, or do you get this feeling sometimes when you are sitting or resting?

Pt: I guess it is mainly when I am up and around.

Dr: Can you tell me, then, how you feel bad when you walk? Try not to say dizzy.
Pt: Well, I feel I'm unsure of myself. I can't trust my walking.
Dr: Does everything around you spin or move, or do you feel like you're spinning?
Pt: No, not exactly.
Dr: Do you feel like you are going to faint?
Pt: I feel like I will fall, not faint.

Notice the mixture of open-ended and directive questions that the physician uses to characterize as precisely as possible what the patient is experiencing. There is much more to find out about this symptom, but from the exchange so far the patient appears to be describing disequilibrium rather than vertigo, presyncope, or lightheadedness.

Another example of the New Brunswick syndrome arose in the following interchange with a patient who came to the doctor because of her cough. Note how the clinician begins with an open-ended question, specifying only that she wishes to hear about the cough, then follows up with Wh questions until the symptom is characterized.

Dr: Tell me about the cough that you've been having.
Pt: It's just worse at night, I can't get no sleep.
Dr: What happens?
Pt: I'm up on three pillows. I'm just miserable, that's all.
Dr: You go up on three pillows to try to prevent the cough?
Pt: Yes.
Dr: How is it miserable?
Pt: Well, if I lay flat I can't breathe, and then I start gasping and gasping for breath, and the only way I can stop is when I sit up and watch TV or something.

The patient in this example actually suffered from congestive heart failure with orthopnea: She became short of breath when she lay flat in bed. She experienced tightness in her chest and a sense of "gasping" for breath that she chose to call "cough." Later in the conversation, the physician learned that she had angina and dyspnea on exertion as well as these nocturnal symptoms.

In this next, longer example, the physician wants to pin down the exact timing of the onset, duration, periodicity, and pattern of chest pain. The physician is concerned that this 62-year-old smoker may have coronary artery disease and knows that only precise symptom description will guide the diagnostic process. Each time the patient gives a somewhat vague statement, the physician follows up with an attempt to clarify.

Pt: . . . and a little bit too fast, it might just be my imagination though, I don't know.

Dr: Uh huh. When did this all start? (Wh question)

Pt: Well, just since the weather has been hot, like it is, you know.

Dr: Several weeks it's been going on, would you say? (clarification)

Pt: Uh huh, just—now the chest pain is not continuous, like, during the day, I don't have to be doing anything, I can just be sitting.

Dr: And where do you feel it? (Wh question)

Pt: It's in here. And like full, just too full, it's fullness in here.

Dr: And then how long does it last when it comes? (Wh question)

Pt: Not too long.

Dr: Minutes, hours? (clarification, laundry list)

Pt: Not hours, just maybe a half hour, or something—you know, it doesn't last.

Dr: Do you do anything that seems to relieve it? (Wh question)

Pt: No, I don't take anything, just sit and be quiet, or either I'll rest. Like, the neighbors, like I told you, were throwing out those old chairs—that recliner, I could use it, so he helped me with it, he put it over the fence and helped me with it into the house and that helps a whole lot. I go in and stretch out on that.

Dr: Uh huh. (minimal facilitator)

Pt: And rest seems to help, when it starts acting up, whenever I could or would be doing around the house, I let it go and just rest.

Dr: Does it sometimes come on while you are doing something? (closed-ended question)

Pt: Yeah, mostly, if I'm doing something like trying to sweep or clean in the house, or something like that.

Dr: How about with walking? (clarification, closed-ended question)

Pt: With walking sometimes, and like mostly. I'll go up to the mall every day and that way I am inside walking and they have benches, I'll sit . . when it starts acting up.

Dr: And then how long does it take to go away once you sit? (Wh question)

Pt: Once I sit, oh, I'll say, half an hour to an hour.

Dr: And it will take a half hour or an hour to go away? (clarification)

Pt: Uh huh.

Dr: Or do you sit for that long even though it's gone before that? (clarification)

Pt: Uh huh. I just sit for that long until it eases.

Dr: And it takes a half hour to an hour for it to ease up? (clarification)

Pt: Uh huh.

Dr: Do you have any other symptoms along with it when you have the pain? (closed-ended question)

Pt: No.

Notice how the clinician in this example tries to establish a pattern of chest pain brought on by exertion and relieved by rest. Perhaps the most critical detail to establish if one suspects coronary artery disease is the length of time it takes for the pain (in this patient, a "fullness" in the chest) to ease with rest. In typical angina, the pain ceases after several minutes or less. This patient is not typical. It is likely that had the response been "Less than 5 minutes" to the question "And then how long does it take to go away once you sit?" the clinician would not have requested further clarification.

Summarization, Confrontation, and Clarification

Summarization is a technique by which the clinician feeds back to the patient the high points of what has been said thus far. Frequent summaries help (1) ensure that the interviewer has the story straight, (2) provide focus, (3) serve as transitions from one topic to another, and (4) keep the interviewer organized. A summary may be as simple as repeating a particularly important statement to see if you have it right, such as: "Okay, as I understand it, the pains you had in 1992 were exactly like the ones you're having now. . . ." In other cases, a brief summary helps you get back on track if the patient is wandering and switching topics, such as: "Okay, we'll get to the cough in a minute, but I need to understand your chest pain better. You said it was like a heavy pressure right in the center of your chest, and it lasted about 5 minutes. . . ."

Summaries are also very useful as transitions from one part of the interview to another. Here is an example of a summary that segues from history of the present illness to the past medical history:

Pt: So that's about how it happened.

Dr: Okay, let me see if I have it straight. You felt perfectly well until 2 days ago when you began to notice an uncomfortable feeling right in the middle here around your belly button, and this has gradually gotten worse, and you are now also having diarrhea. (Patient nods.) OK, I think I understand pretty well what's been going on the last 2 days. How about in the past, have you had any problems with your health in the past?

Sometimes as you try to summarize, you note discrepancies in the story; and because you want to know exactly what happened, it is usually necessary to point out those discrepancies. When you do this, you are using **confrontation**. This rather dramatic word arose from interviewing techniques in psychotherapy. It has connotations of pointing out falsehoods, rationalizations, or neurotic conflicts, and in its everyday usage often implies opposing sides. In the medical interview, however, confrontation is simply an attempt to clarify inconsistent statements; you heard one thing and now it appears the patient is describing the experience differently, or contradicting an earlier statement. Which version is right? For example:

Dr: Now let me see if I can understand this. You said before that you were coughing up some bloody stuff with that heavy cough last year. But just now you said, when this cough developed yesterday, it was the first time you ever saw blood come up. Did I misunderstand you?

In other words, confrontation is a device to clarify the data. You say what you heard, but ask for more detail, perhaps to resolve ambiguities in the story, as in the example of our earlier patient with chest pain.

A FEW EXAMPLES

Here are three examples of beginnings of interviews. In each case, we have labeled the clinician's statements or questions with the technique being used. Note the importance, in this part of the interview, of social greetings, nondirective questions, minimal facilitators, clarification, and summarization.

Example 1

Dr: Okay, hello again. I'm Dr. Block. Tell me what I can do for you today. (social greeting, nondirective question)

Pt: Well, I have a terrible vaginal itch, and I don't know whether it's the vaginitis or whether it's the urine, urinary tract infection. My regular doctor treated me for vaginitis.

Dr: That was Dr. Hill? (clarification, facilitation)

Pt: Uh huh. Then I got, um, a urinary tract infection and then the vaginitis came back. But during the whole ordeal, I've never got any relief.

Dr: During the treatment for the vaginitis, during the treatment for the urinary tract infection, you still had this terrible itch? (summary, clarification)

Example 2

Dr: Good morning. (social greeting)

Pt: (Patient is seated on end of exam table) Good morning.

Dr: Why don't you have a seat back over here, and we can talk a little bit first. Tell me why you came today. (attending to the patient's comfort, nondirective question)

Pt: Um, to get my blood pressure checked.

Dr: To get your blood pressure checked? What do you know about your blood pressure? (reflective response, nondirective question with topic specified)

Pt: Well, I have heard various things over the past couple of years, really, that it has been high, and um . . .

Dr: For several years? (clarification and facilitation)

Pt: (Nods) And I went about, oh, it was quite a while ago, maybe 5 or 6 months ago to the health center, um, and the doctor told me it was high, but he could not treat me until I lost approximately 38 pounds, so I haven't been able to take the weight off and I was kind of, well, he did not give me any special diet to follow or you know, what I should cut out of my diet, and I was very discouraged by it, so when I went to the emergency room because I cut my finger, um, the nurse told me that my blood pressure was very high and I should have it checked, and since I don't have a family doctor, she suggested I come here.

Example 3

Dr: It's nice to see you again. What brings you here today? (social greeting, open-ended question)

Pt: Doctor, I'm not well.

Dr: I take it you have not been feeling really well for a while. (summary based on previous knowledge of this patient)

Pt: No, well, I haven't been feeling very good for about the last, oh, I'd say about a week, about a week now.

Dr: Uh huh. (facilitation)

Pt: About a week now, I haven't been feeling good.

Dr: What have you noticed? (nondirective question)

Pt: Oh, some soreness in here right through here, and some pain in my arm and a, a, a strangulating feeling right in here and a burning in the, in the middle, right here and a burning in my throat, a little bit, and dizzy—I felt real dizzy when I was on the scale out there, you know, and I called you and the nurse, and she helped me and I wasn't real bad and you know, I told her to open a window and she said first "do you want me to open a window" and I said "yeah and I want to get near the air."

Dr: Does that help? (clarification)

Pt: Oh yeah.

CHALLENGES TO ELICITING THE CHIEF COMPLAINT AND PRESENT ILLNESS

The patient's style of speaking may present challenges in getting a coherent story. The profoundly depressed patient may not have enough energy to give a detailed, logical story, whereas the anxious and talkative patient may embellish his or her story with unnecessary details. Some patients are so reticent that you find yourself asking a series of narrow, closed-ended questions until the interview comes to a distressing stop. Other patients have so much to say that you feel as though you are losing control in a confusing quagmire. You worry that, when the interview is over, you may know a lot about the patient but very little about the illness.

The Reticent Patient

THE PROBLEM

The reticent patient simply says nothing, or almost nothing. When only a limited amount of information is needed (e.g., a patient with an acute laceration or a sore throat), this may not be a problem. There are other times, however, when lack of detail seriously compromises history taking, such as for the patient on p. 55 with chest pain, in whom a detailed and unambiguous history is essential for making the diagnosis.

THE REMEDY

The trick here is to guide the reticent patient without asking leading questions; sometimes one way of asking an open-ended question works where another way does not. Consider this example:

Dr: Can you tell me what the problem is?
Pt: Uh, that's what I came to see you about, Doc.
Dr: What have your symptoms been?
Pt: Tired, awful tired.

It almost appears as though the interview will come to an end with the first question, but the interviewer simply asks another open-ended question that, this time around, elicits the chief complaint. A "laundry list" or menu is another useful technique. This interview went on:

Dr: Can you tell me more about it?
Pt: No, just tired.

> **Dr:** When you say tired, do you mean a feeling of not being rested or a feeling of weakness in your muscles? Or do you have trouble doing things you used to do because you get short of breath?
>
> **Pt:** That's it, Doc, just not rested.

The physician uses a menu to clarify the symptom without leading the patient. Notice the difference between asking the patient to choose from several possibilities and raising the same possibilities in a sequence of yes/no questions. In the latter case, you can never be sure that the patient is not simply saying what he or she thinks you want to hear.

Patients may be reticent because of depression, dementia (simply cannot remember the symptoms), anxiety, denial, a taciturn personality style, or cultural distance from the physician. Some patients expect to be interrogated like witnesses. These persons may have trouble with an open directive like "Tell me what happened," and respond better to more structure: "Tell me what happened first" and then, "What happened next?" They may need frequent reminders demonstrating your open, relaxed attitude, such as "It is important for me to know exactly how you felt when that happened—tell me as best you can."

The Patient Who Rambles

THE PROBLEM

Some patients embellish their problems with numerous seemingly unrelated details. In other settings such persons might be considered exquisite storytellers, but you have a limited amount of time for the interview, and entertainment is not your goal. Sometimes the details seem connected to the story, as with our patient on p. 46; at other times it is difficult to see any connection at all. At times the details are related to the medical history but are unnecessary, such as the patient who has an attack of diarrhea and describes in great detail his or her attempt to find a bathroom.

THE REMEDY

The trick is to direct the patient back to the task at hand without appearing to be rude or disinterested. One way to do this is to acknowledge your own confusion and feeling of being lost in the details, as well as your need to accomplish the task at hand. Most patients accept this kind of direction very well. For example, you might say to the patient with diarrhea:

Dr: It certainly sounds as though you had a hard time with that episode; since our time is limited, though, perhaps you can tell me more about the diarrhea itself. Tell me what it was like.

In this instance the physician uses a summary statement ("sounds as though you had a hard time") and a reminder of time constraints, followed by a question that directs the interview back to the characterization of the illness.

In an earlier example on p. 46, an interviewer's open-ended question ("Now what can I do for you, Mrs. P?") leads to a deluge of disconnected information that would leave most clinicians feeling totally bewildered and wondering where to go next. Although this patient may have stated most of her medical history in one fell swoop, it is difficult to sort it out. Many clinicians are reluctant to ask open-ended questions because they fear receiving precisely this kind of rambling response. In reality such responses are infrequent. When they do occur, it is best to acknowledge your confusion and try to direct the patient to one topic at a time. One possible reply might be:

Dr: Okay, I'm getting a bit confused. Let's see if we can take one problem at a time. You mentioned tiredness even though you seem to get a lot of sleep. Other than the hot flashes, is there anything else that seems to wake you up at night?

Either during or after the interview, you will have a chance to think about why the patient talks this way. Among the causes are anxiety, loneliness, histrionic personality style, thought disorder, or a particular set of beliefs about how symptoms and events are related. Sometimes this kind of response is simply the person's conversational style, which is less appropriate in the context of a professional relationship than it is in a social interaction. Sometimes the associations are so bizarre that you must consider psychiatric illness as the cause.

The Vague Patient

THE PROBLEM

With the vague patient, the interviewer cannot figure out exactly what the patient is describing. You may wonder whether the symptom itself is vague or whether it is simply the patient's description of it that is vague. Some sensations are difficult to describe, such as dizziness or poorly localized abdominal pain. When you know the patient, it is easier to judge the source of the problem. The patient who, in the past, has always given a precise history is probably experiencing a vague sensation, whereas a patient who has a vague conversational style may well have a precise symptom that simply requires more work to translate into medically useful words.

THE REMEDY

One technique for the vague patient is to provide a choice of useful descriptors without leading the patient. For example, you might use a menu such as, "Was the pain sharp, dull, or burning?" or "Was it all over, or in just one place, or did it move from place to place?" Alternatively, you can ask if it resembles a symptom with which both the patient and physician are familiar, such as (for lower abdominal or pelvic pain in a woman), "Does it feel anything like menstrual cramps?" Another approach is to ask the patient if he or she has ever felt anything like this particular symptom before, and then to ask, "What's different about it this time?" To find the location of a vague symptom, you can ask the patient to point to where it hurts.

The following two examples illustrate vague openings. In the first example, the physician simply indicates that vague terminology such as "cold" or "flu" (". . . tell me more about what you mean") is unacceptable, and the patient begins to describe the symptoms in more detail. The patient in the second example does not respond to simple requests for more precision.

Example 1

Dr: What can I do for you?

Pt: (Clearing throat) I think I've got, um, a cold or flu or something . . . yesterday I felt terrible, so I feel I just need some kind of a prescription. . . .

Dr: OK. Tell me, you say you have a cold; tell me more about what you mean.

Pt: Um (Clearing throat) fatigue is the most. . . .

Dr: Fatigue?

Pt: Just kind of drained.

Dr: Aha.

Pt: Kind of scratchy throat, not really sore. Ah, a lot of drainage. . . .

Dr: Coughing?

Pt: A little bit, but not getting anything up.

Dr: Just sort of dry?

Pt: Dry coughing, I don't feel as though there's anything collected down there yet. And, that's another thing that worries me, having had a history of asthma, I have a fear of bronchitis.

Example 2

Pt: Well, doctor, well, I got the dizziness, I'm getting more, looks like I'm, looks like I'm getting tired and more tired, I go up the steps and I just, just like dizziness, I, I go like this, I just go dark, I, and I can't see.

Dr: What do you mean by dizziness?

Pt: When I go up the steps and when I get up in the morning, I got that dizziness again, I'm just falling back.

Dr: What happens to you when you're dizzy?

Pt: Well, when, when I drink water, if I drink cold water, that's when I get it, then I start having chills, I get real cold, just like I'm shaking.

Dr: But how do you feel when you're dizzy?

Pt: I just go back, like this, and then sometimes I, I can't see, I, I have to close my eyes like that and then open my eyes up like that and I still can't just like. . . .

In the second example, we are left wondering whether the patient's description is vague or the symptom is vague. The physician could have taken the tack of asking: "Tell me what you mean, but try not to use the word 'dizzy.'" Another possibility would be to provide a menu:

Dr: When you say dizziness, is it a feeling that you may pass out or that you may lose your balance?

Pt: No, not exactly.

Dr: Could you describe it as a spinning sensation as though you or the room is moving, or is it more of a lightheadedness?

Pt: That's it, lightheaded, just lightheaded.

Whether the patient is reticent, verbose, rambling, or vague, the clinician's goal is to obtain a story that is clear, internally consistent, logical, and not fictional. Most patients desire these features as well but may not necessarily share with the physician the same criteria for judging them. Your first approach is to clarify, teach, or demonstrate the kind of story that will be helpful. If this approach does not work, you are probably faced with one or more of three issues:

- The patient's basic personality style, perhaps stressed by the illness, interferes with telling an adequate story.

- Some strong emotion or affect gets in the way of the patient's telling a clear, logical story.

- The patient's beliefs are sufficiently different from yours that a story that appears incoherent is actually quite logical once you understand the basic premises from which the patient reasons.

We examine these issues in Chapters 10 and 14. We conclude the present chapter with a summary of techniques that help you obtain accurate and precise data during the early part of the medical history.

S U M M A R Y : Chief Complaint and History of the Present Illness

In this chapter we discussed, first, how to set the stage and get started:

- Establish a sense of privacy for the interview.
- Introduce yourself appropriately and establish a contract.
- Maintain an attentive body position.
- Minimize distractions.
- Take notes, but maintain enough eye contact so as not to "lose" the patient.
- Use language the patient can understand.

The next step is to obtain the chief complaint:

- Record the chief complaint in the patient's own words.
- Consider the possibility that the iatrotropic stimulus, or actual reason for coming, is different from the ostensible chief complaint.

With regard to the history of the present illness, we presented the following facilitative techniques:

- Move from the general to the specific, using open-ended questions to introduce each topic.
- Use nonverbal encouragment, like silence and head nods; and minimal facilitators, like mirrors, paraphrases, and saying "Uh huh," "And?" or "Yes?"
- Proceed to Wh questions to characterize symptoms.
- Employ menus or direct questions when necessary for specification or efficiency.
- Strive for interchangeable responses to show that you are listening and encourage disclosure of accurate information about thoughts and feelings.
- Avoid leading questions that reveal the answer you expect or desire, or multiple questions that confuse the patient.

- Give the patient time to answer in his or her own words.
- Clarify and maintain direction for both the patient and yourself by using summaries, clarification, and, when needed, confrontation.

Among the challenges to obtaining a good narrative are various interactive styles, including those involving patients who are reticent, vague, or rambling. We illustrated various techniques that may help you overcome these challenges.

References

1. Beckman HB, Frankel RM. The effect of physician behavior on the collection of data. *Ann Intern Med* 1984; 101:692–696.
2. Bass LW, Cohen RL. Ostensible versus actual reasons for seeking pediatric attention: Another look at the parental ticket of admission. *Pediatrics* 1982; 70:870–874.
3. Feinstein AR. *Clinical Judgment.* Baltimore, Williams & Wilkins, 1967.
4. White J, Levinson W, Roter D. "Oh, by the way . . ." The closing moments of the medical visit. *J Gen Intern Med* 1994; 9:24–28.
5. Reilly BM. *Practical Strategies in Outpatient Medicine.* Philadelphia, WB Saunders, 1984.

Suggested Readings

Lipkin M Jr. The medical interview and related skills. In: Branch WT (Ed.) *Office Practice of Medicine.* Philadelphia, WB Saunders, 1987, pp. 1287–1306.

Platt FW. *Conversation Failure. Case Studies in Doctor-Patient Communication.* Tacoma, WA, Life Sciences Press, 1992.

Platt FW. *Conversation Repair. Case Studies in Doctor-Patient Communication.* Boston, Little, Brown, 1995.

CHAPTER 4

Transforming Experience into Memory

• • •

OTHER ACTIVE PROBLEMS, PAST MEDICAL HISTORY, AND FAMILY HISTORY

To hold a true belief about an event in one's past experience is not sufficient for remembering it. There is still a distinctive factor lacking . . . Now it sometimes happens that a belief . . . transforms itself into a memory.

A. J. Ayer, *The Problem of Knowledge*

Once you have elicited the chief complaint and present illness, other parts of the history, although tedious at first, are, in a sense, easier because they deal with structured data and specific questions about predetermined topics. The trick is to emphasize the relevant features of past health and medical care experiences without getting too overwhelmed with a mass of detail. Feinstein[1] has cautioned us to avoid the "Scylla of overdirection" and the "Charybdis of digression." By this he means the ability to keep your inquiry open-ended enough to avoid missing the important events without getting bogged down in endless details about unimportant events.

This chapter and the two that follow cover parts of the medical interview that fill in the total picture of your patient's health and illness experience. These aspects of the interview provide important details that enhance your evaluation of, and response to, the person's current illness. In this chapter, we discuss the search for other active problems, past medical history, and family history. These components provide you with information about the context or setting in which the illness occurs, including the previous state of the patient's health, as well as the presence of risk factors that have implications for both the current diagnosis and the prevention of future ills.

OTHER ACTIVE PROBLEMS

You have just made it through the history of the present illness, working hard to maintain the narrative thread (what happened first, what happened next) without getting sidetracked by distractions, such as a too-early preoccupation with what the diagnosis is. You begin to build the themes of the interview: what the story of the illness is, who the patient is, how the interview is going. You progressively narrow your focus to delineate a single problem or condition that you hope will explain the patient's symptoms and findings. At this point, however, you should step back and ask yourself: What am I missing here? What else could be going on with this patient? In other words, what are the patient's **other active problems** (OAPs)?

In today's medicine, patients often have a number of chronic conditions that may impact upon their current distress. The notion of a singular "present illness" that is quite distinct from "past medical history" is no longer tenable: a patient who comes to the emergency room because of fever and productive cough may at the same time be under treatment for diabetes, hypertension, coronary heart disease, and osteoporosis. In this case, the patient has several active medical problems, any of which may contribute to, or must be considered in responding to, his or her current syndrome. Thus, it is crucial to differentiate these problems from the traditional items in past medical history (e.g., appendectomy in 1976, motor vehicle accident in 1984, an allergy to ampicillin noted in 1989).

The search for OAPs may be accomplished by asking nondirective questions at the end of the present illness segment of the interview. For example,

- "Okay, I think I've gotten the story straight so far. Has anything else been bothering you?"
- "Can you think of other symptoms or problems that you've had recently?"
- "Do you have any other illnesses that have been acting up lately, or that you see a doctor for?"

In this way other problems that relate to, or influence, the present illness may be uncovered early, thereby avoiding last-minute surprises during the review of systems. A patient may be admitted to the hospital with pneumonia but may also suffer from chronic renal failure, diabetes, and hypertension. These chronic illnesses are also current problems and clearly affect the situation at hand.

Another good screening question for OAPs is, "What medications do you take?" Regardless of what the patient responds to this, always broaden your inquiry to include any regularly used drugs, such as oral contraceptives (which the patient may not consider a *medication*), aspirin, cold preparations, pain relievers, and over-the-counter laxatives. Remember also to ask about vitamins or mineral (e.g., iron or calcium) tablets. Because many people consider these "natural" products and not medications, they may not mention them unless specifically asked.

Here is an example of an interview in which a 62-year-old retired metal worker came to the physician's office for a complete check-up "because I've never really had one." The physician picks up at the end of the present illness segment:

Dr: Okay, so the main concern you have, aside from wanting a check-up, is this pain in your left side. Are you having any other problems with your health?

Pt: No, nothing really. As I said, the main thing is to establish a relationship with a family doctor.

Dr: Okay, that's good. Let me find out a little more about you. Do you take any medications?

Pt: Yeah, well, Dr. Gold has had me on that Vasoretic for a few years for my pressure.

Notice how this patient, like many people, requires repeated open-ended prompts to reveal continuing and obviously important details about his health. What is going on here? Certainly, the patient is not trying to hide the fact that he takes medication for hypertension; indeed, it may have become so routine to him that he doesn't initially label it as a health "problem." Most likely, the physician would have stumbled on this information later in the interview during an extensive past medical history or an exhaustive review of systems, but it is an important feature to know up-front: in a routine check-up, chronic hypertension makes a difference.

The past medical history sometimes also presents opportunities to explore OAPs. If the patient reports serious, chronic, or ill-defined symptoms in the past, it is a good idea to ask if these or similar symptoms are occurring now.

THE PAST MEDICAL HISTORY

You can begin your inquiry with a general question:

- "How has your health been in the past?"
- "Tell me about any serious illnesses you have had in the past, starting from when you were a child."
- "Now I'd like to ask you about any illnesses or medical problems you've had in the past. How has your health been?"
- "Okay, I think I understand what's been happening in the past few weeks, how about your health in the past?"

Patients may respond in general terms such as, "I've always been sickly," or "Well, I used to have stomach problems," or, alternatively, begin to discuss particular symptoms. You should focus the inquiry on discrete episodes that caused substantial disability or a difference in the usual health pattern, and attempt to determine the diagnosis they, or their physicians, have given to these illnesses.

You should never simply assume that a diagnosis the patient relates is, in fact, the correct medical diagnosis. For example, a patient might tell you that he or she has had "four or five heart attacks" in the past when, in fact, the patient has never suffered an acute myocardial infarction; this problem arises because the term "heart attack" means different things to different people. A good question to ask is, "What exactly were your symptoms that made the doctor think that?"

There is no point, however, in trying to confirm every item of the past history by grilling the patient on obscure details. Your time and energy and those of the patient are limited. Here is how one physician, who himself became a patient, expressed his feelings about being asked "ancient history":

> It's bad enough that I don't know all my family's medical diseases or what my grandparents, whom I never knew, died of, but I begin to feel positively stupid when at the mature age of 44 I do not know whether as an infant I had measles or chickenpox. I may do a little better with more recent conditions, but the feeling sinks again when it comes to medications I've taken that have given me trouble. "Those little red pills" seems an insufficient answer, and the recording physician's dubious look does not help much. . . . By this point in the interview, when I am asked questions about the specific timing and location of my varying symptoms, I begin to answer with a specificity born more of desperation than accuracy.[2]

Adult patients frequently have one or more chronic illnesses, and each of these may have had several exacerbations or have required hospitalizations at different times. They may or may not be relevant to the current illness. Consider a patient who has rapidly progressive congestive heart failure symptoms, in the absence of hypertension or known ischemic heart disease, and who was referred to a medical faculty member. Because the patient had a dilated heart, predominance of severe right-sided heart failure, and symptoms that appeared to begin rather suddenly, the referring doctor thought the patient might have a congestive cardiomyopathy. However, the past medical history revealed quite frequent episodes of "acute bronchitis" and "pneumonia," and the search for OAP also yielded the information that the patient had a chronic "cigarette cough," usually producing sputum each morning. The patient was found to have chronic obstructive pulmonary disease and cor pulmonale. Neither she nor her physician had related her recurrent lung problems and cigarette smoking to the illness at hand. When the consultant made this connection, it became clear that the present illness really extended much further into the past than was initially thought to have been the case.

After you acquire general information about the person's past health, you fill in important categories of past medical history (as shown in Table 4–1). Old records can and should be obtained when, on the basis of your evaluation, you believe the information will be relevant to caring for the patient. A couple of pointers on specificity:

- **Dates.** The exact date or year of an illness, if remote, is generally not important. Inquiry that is too precise will lead both to frustration and to falsely precise answers ("specificity born of desperation"). A "hysterectomy in the early 1970s" is usually adequate; it does not matter whether it was 1972 or 1973.

- **Allergies.** You should clarify what your patient means by the term "allergy." A person may tell you he is allergic to flu shots because, after having one, he had several colds that winter, or another may tell you that she is allergic to aspirin because it gives her stomach discomfort. The first case is a personal attribution of a poor outcome, and the second case illustrates a side effect rather than a true allergy to aspirin. Be sure to ask specifically about allergies to medications.

Here is an example of a past medical history obtained from a 39-year-old woman at her first office visit for evaluation of headaches. She was found

TABLE 4–1 PAST MEDICAL HISTORY

Serious illnesses, beginning in childhood
Hospitalizations
Surgical procedures
Accidents or injuries
Obstetrical history (women)
Allergies
Current medications
Immunizations

to have elevated blood pressure. Note the ease with which the clinician prepares the patient for each new topic:

Dr: Okay, let's talk about your past health. Did you have any unusual childhood illnesses, rheumatic fever, scarlet fever, diphtheria?

Pt: Bronchitis.

Dr: Bronchitis. What do you mean by bronchitis?

Pt: Well, I'm not sure. That's what my mother told me. I guess I used to get sick a lot when I was a kid.

Dr: Were you ever hospitalized? Any serious illnesses or operations?

Pt: Uh huh.

Dr: What have you been hospitalized for?

Pt: When I've had D & Cs done, and I had my appendix out with part of my ovary.

Dr: Part of your ovary came out and . . .?

Pt: Well, I have a history of cysts growing on my ovaries.

Dr: Were you followed by a gynecologist?

Pt: Yes, Dr. Smith here in town.

Dr: Now, you mentioned you have two children. Any problems with your pregnancies or with childbirth?

Pt: With my little girl, yes. I had a lot of water, plus I had a bladder infection.

Dr: Did you have high blood pressure with that?

Pt: No, but I was sick a lot, nauseated a lot. It was like morning sickness but I had it for 8 months with her.

Dr: Doctor put you to bed at all?

Pt: No.

Dr: Any other hospitalizations, any other medical problems in the past that you had that you can remember?

Pt: No, just the D & Cs and the children and that one operation I had.

Dr: Do you have any known allergies?

Pt: I am allergic to goldenrod.

Dr: To what?

Pt: Goldenrod. Wool. I have hay fever. Anything like flowers—I get around them, I constantly sneeze my head off or get stuffed up. Roses, stuff like that. Right now, I'm having a time because we went up to the lake and we have a lot of goldenrod growing wild.

Dr: Do you take anything for it?

This is an example of a fairly typical and complete past history that demonstrates how "old" news is relevant to the present problems. Notice how the physician asks exactly what the patient means by bronchitis. Although the patient is not sure, she later reports symptoms of allergy; symptoms of allergy plus a childhood history of bronchitis suggest atopy, with the bronchitis perhaps representing episodes of childhood asthma. The patient has now "outgrown" her asthma but still has an atopic disposition, as evidenced by the hay fever symptoms. The physician also uncovers the history of fluid retention during pregnancy. This symptom could have represented toxemia, possibly of relevance to her hypertension now. Notice how the doctor asks specifically if the patient had high blood pressure. He also tries to determine if she was treated for hypertension without realizing it by asking, "Doctor put you to bed at all?" Another way to ask would be, "How was that treated?" The question regarding whether the patient takes anything for her hay fever is relevant for at least three reasons: (1) to avoid the embarrassment of recommending something the patient has already tried; (2) to help ascertain symptom severity; and (3) to learn if medications that can raise blood pressure in susceptible persons were used.

Our final example is that of a patient who was being seen for back pain and reported a past history of phlebitis. What follows is the physician's search for evidence that he did, indeed, have phlebitis:

Pt: But I have more trouble in my left leg than I do in the right leg, normally with this phlebitis that I had.

Dr: Were you ever admitted to the hospital for phlebitis and given intravenous medicines?

Pt: It's so long ago I don't remember.

Dr: Did you ever take a blood thinner?

Pt: Yes, Coumadin.

Dr: You were on Coumadin at one time. Did they ever do any x-ray studies of your legs with a dye? Did they ever put a . . .

Pt: I had the fibrinogen test. I had a series of tests.

Dr: Fibrinogen scans . . .

Pt: Yes, I had a series of tests done.

Dr: Did they ever do a venogram?

Pt: I don't know what that is.

Dr: You would remember it. A venogram is where they put a needle into a vein in your foot, and they inject a dye.

Pt: No, they didn't do that.

Dr: So you haven't had a venogram done.

Pt: I was taking iodine and had to take the iodine every day and come to the hospital every day for a month. I think that was the fibrinogen test.

Dr: The fibrinogen scan. Did you ever have, I imagine you would have had, something called a Doppler study.

Pt: I don't remember.

Dr: Or IPG, that's where they use sound waves to look for clots in the legs.

Pt: Is it a machine?

Dr: Yes.

Pt: I was on a machine in the emergency room one night.

Dr: On a machine for . . .

Pt: . . . for phlebitis.

Dr: Checking your legs, or do you mean one of the IV machines?

Pt: No, it wasn't IV.

Dr: Is it a machine where they ran a little microphone-like thing?

Pt: No, they put little things on like they're going to take your blood pressure. They put them on my legs.

Dr: So they were studying blood clots. So, you have been on . . . were you only on the Coumadin one time?

Pt: Twice.

Dr: Twice. And you were hospitalized both times?

Pt: No, I wasn't hospitalized.

Dr: You weren't. You were never hospitalized before you were put on Coumadin.

Pt: No. I was in the emergency room and then I went to the doctor's office.

Dr: And they put you on Coumadin. You never had any heparin.

Pt: No, I didn't have heparin. I had Coumadin. The little white pills.

Dr: Right. That's interesting.

FAMILY HISTORY

The **family history** is the systematic exploration of the presence or absence of any illness in the patient's family that may have an impact on the diagnosis of the patient's illness, or that influences the patient's health or risk of future disease.

First, what illnesses and conditions are relevant? They include:

- Frankly hereditary diseases, such as sickle cell anemia or dyslipo-proteinemias

- Familial illnesses, such as coronary artery disease, adult-onset diabetes mellitus, or carcinoma of the breast, in which genetic factors play a significant role

- Family traits, such as short stature

- Illnesses such as manic-depressive disorder or alcoholism, which may not only be familial, but also profoundly affect the patient's environment

- Current illnesses in the family that *may* suggest an infectious process or toxic exposure in the environment

Second, what do we mean by "family"? To determine the risk of hereditary disease, we generally mean the patient's parents, siblings, and children; of somewhat lesser importance, the patient's grandparents, cousins, aunts, and uncles. The spouse is a vital member of the patient's family but is of no importance to familial disease. However, in dealing with contagious disease and toxic exposures, we might expand the concept of "family" to include the whole household, perhaps in this instance even broadening to include the patient's place of work.

The family history always enriches our understanding of the patient, whether in making a diagnosis or in managing the illness, but because time and energy are limited, the potentially enormous amount of information must be tailored to the specific situation. How much we want to know depends on the patient, the type of problem, and the ability of the patient to give the information. For example, a family history of breast cancer is obviously of less relevance to a 10-year-old boy with tonsillitis than to a 45-year-old woman with a breast mass. A seriously ill patient may have a very relevant family history but be too sick to give it. This might be the situation, say, in a seriously ill patient with an acute myocardial infarction whose father died of a heart attack at age 44; the family history can wait until the patient feels well enough to remember and discuss the details.

Good ways to start the routine family history are:

- "Are there any illnesses that seem to run in your family?"
- "Has anyone in your family been seriously ill?"
- "How about your parents? Children?"
- "Has anyone in your family ever had anything like the symptoms you are having now?"
- "Has anyone in your family had heart attacks?"

In the case of an acute, possibly contagious illness, it is helpful to begin:

- "Has anyone else at home or work been sick lately?"
- "Have you come into contact with anyone who has similar symptoms?"

Here is an excerpt of a routine family history that will give you a sense of the flow of this part of the medical interview. Notice how the physician first introduces the new subject area (a transition) and then goes on with a specific question:

Dr: Okay. I think I understand the symptoms. Now I'd like to find out a little about your family. How about your parents, are they still living?

Pt: They're deceased.

Dr: Do you recall what they passed away from?

Pt: My mother had a heart attack 2 months ago.

Dr: How old was she at that time?

Pt: 63, I think.

Dr: How about your father?

Pt: About 7 years ago.

Dr: What did he pass away from?

Pt: Lung cancer.

Dr: How old was he?

Pt: Oh, I'd say 57.

Dr: Brothers or sisters?

Pt: Yes, I have nine brothers—I mean I have five brothers and three sisters.

Dr: Do they have medical problems that you are aware of ?

Pt: No.

Dr: Is there any history of high blood pressure in the family?

Pt: My mother.

Dr: Your mother, okay. How about diabetes?

Pt: No.

The physician begins with a general question about problems or illnesses, then follows up with some specific yes/no questions about illnesses that one tends to see in families, such as hypertension and diabetes, or illnesses of particular relevance to this patient, who has hypertension.

But we observe something else here. Notice that the patient's mother is **recently** deceased. The physician here faces a choice about how to proceed, given this information. Should she explore the patient's feelings, or continue with the family history? In this instance, the physician proceeds with the history and this approach appears to be useful. Had the patient's mother died at an advanced age after increasing illness or disability, the physician would expect the patient to feel differently than if she died suddenly at a relatively young age. A potential problem here is that the physician accepts the stated diagnosis of "heart attack" and learns little more. There are many possibilities: Was it a sudden event? Were there many previous attacks? Was she sickly for years, perhaps with rheumatic heart disease and a final deadly "attack"? And what of the resulting effects on this person—the patient—with a sickly mother? The physician will, later in the interview, return to her recent loss and deal with it more effectively and compassionately. Information about diseases in the family has social, as well as medical, dimensions. Everyone has feelings about his or her close relatives, especially parents and children. There is no way to avoid this; we can, however, acknowledge it, be prepared for it, and deal with it in a compassionate way during the interview.

Knowledge about family history shapes the patient's beliefs and worries about health, health risks, and current symptoms. A patient with chest pain may believe that she has a bad heart like her mother, even though she is young and suffering from a totally different type of problem. A patient approaching the same age at which a parent died may have special concerns about his or her own health. Consider this family history in a 41-year-old woman who came because "it's been a while since I had a good checkup":

Dr: Your parents still living?

Pt: My father is living. My mother died when she was 42.

Dr: How is your father? Is he in good health?

Pt: Uh huh.

Dr: How old is he?

Pt: He was born in 1926.

Dr: So he's 71.

Pt: Yes.

Dr: Any brothers or sisters?

Pt: Two sisters. Both are in good health as far as I know. I don't keep very good contact with them, because I live here and they live out of state.

Dr: Any medical problems? You said there are some medical problems that run in your family. What are they again?

Pt: My mother had a bad heart. Most of it is in my mother's family. Like my grandmother died, she had cancer. She had diabetes too. When my mother died, she had had a plastic valve put in, then slowly deteriorated. She had sclerosis of the liver and a bad heart. She lived about a year after she had the plastic valve put in.

A woman who dies at the age of 42 after having an artificial valve probably had rheumatic, or possibly congenital, heart disease. Although there is some chance that the daughter may suffer from a similar problem, of more relevance is the daughter's beliefs about the matter. Note that she is 41 years old and her mother died at age 42. If she is found to have no signs of heart disease, it will be important to reassure her that her symptoms are totally unrelated to what went on with her mother.

Even the most straightforward questions sometimes lead to double-edged answers:

Dr: You said you've been pregnant five times?

Pt: Yes.

Dr: Do your children live at home with you?

Pt: Yes.

Dr: Five of them?

Pt: Yes.

Dr: How old are they?

Pt: 20, 15, 13, 10.

Dr: That's four children.

Pt: Oh, I lost one.

Dr: Did he die of disease?

Pt: No, he died—he had a little growth on his eye and he died in surgery.

The physician dedicated to using a mechanical set of family history questions could have simply ignored the fact that she gave only four ages. While the death of her child seems to have no strictly "medical" bearing whatever, a parent who has lost a child will certainly have feelings attached to the memory of the event and also may have negative feelings about the medical system which, she may believe, caused her child's death.

In some cases, discussion of family history may cause the patient to become anxious. In asking about family diseases, you imply that they may be related to the patient's current medical problem. It is helpful to be reassuring and to emphasize the "routine" nature of the inquiry. Here is an example of a physician who stumbles on anxiety-provoking information in asking a routine family history question:

Dr: Yeah, Okay. Very good. Now your mother and father, what did they . . . Are they still alive?

Pt: Um, my mother is alive, my . . .

Dr: Age?

Notice how the physician hesitates over the initial question, realizing that the first thing he needs to know is if the parents are living; then, barely listening to the response, the doctor asks another question. The dialogue continues:

Pt: She is 64.

Dr: She have any illnesses you know of?

Pt: Uh . . .

Dr: Heart disease, lung disease, anything?

Pt: No, nothing of that sort; she's had a well-known skin cancer and uh, and she seems to have a recurring, it's a problem with her back, but actually it's a nerve that has to be blocked every once in a while.

Dr: Okay. Your father?

Pt: I never really knew that much about my father, but as I understand it he died of a cerebral hemorrhage.

Dr: How old was he?

Pt: Oh, he must have been in his early 40s.

Dr: Was an autopsy done or anything to find out . . .

> **Pt:** There was so little . . . there was a bad occurrence, bad divorce between our mother and father when I was real young and I never saw him after age 9 months really. So I'm very hazy on the particulars of this.

The physician here stumbles on two kinds of loaded information: (1) that the father died of a cerebral hemorrhage at about the same age the patient is now; and (2) that the patient does not know much about it because of a "bad occurrence." The physician ignores the "bad occurrence" and goes after a possible cause of the hemorrhage, congenital berry aneurysm being relevant here because this condition can be hereditary.

> **Dr:** But nobody knew whether it was traumatic; did he get hit or anything?
> **Pt:** I don't know the details, to tell you the truth. He had, well, I just don't really know enough to talk about it.
> **Dr:** Cerebral hemorrhage at a young age would be an unusual thing. No other causes being known.
> **Pt:** I could find out more, my mother may know more about it.
> **Dr:** If she knew, it would be important to you—if she would know, for instance, if he had an aneurysm in his brain that burst, which is one of the ways you can have a cerebral hemorrhage at a young age. I think that would be very important, for instance, for your general health information, so perhaps you can find out. Okay? Do you know anything more in terms of other problems?

Note the physician's graphic description of "an aneurysm in his brain that burst" and the statement that this "would be very important to you" while quickly moving on to "other problems." The patient, whom we first met on p. 22, now goes on to talk about the "painful subject" while the physician completely ignores the affective content of the interview.

> **Pt:** Well, my understanding is, the context of this, that my mother was raised in the Catholic church and divorce was a terrible scandal in her mind, and she tried to forget about it as quickly as she could. It's such a painful subject that there was never any discussion about who he was and so forth. And as a consequence, all I've really heard are niblets, and one of the things I understand is that he was an alcoholic, or at least had a problem with alcohol, but really caused my mother a lot of problems. So, I don't know if that would be a complicating factor in terms of aneurysm or not.
> **Dr:** Not that I know of. How about brothers and sisters?

Pt: I have one full natural brother and then four half brothers.
Dr: Any medical problems in any of them that you know of?
Pt: No.

This example demonstrates a doctor's insensitivity to the patient's feelings and self-disclosure. It also shows that, by pursuing an item of family history, the doctor can increase the patient's anxiety and raise new questions in the patient's mind about his or her own health. A person who tells you that his sister had breast cancer, that his father (who smoked two packs of cigarettes per day for all of his adult life) developed lung cancer, or that his uncle (an asbestos worker) died from mesothelioma may feel that he is at high risk for developing the same diseases, or at least some form of cancer. The more you press for details, the more your patient may feel that there is a connection with his or her present illness. Such a patient who does not have the environmental exposures may need reassurance that he or she is not at special personal risk.

Another source of anxiety arises from the psychologic bias called **availability.** An unusual illness that happens to occur in a family member is highly visible and "available" to the patient. Therefore, it has a greater impact on his or her fears than we, as medical practitioners, might feel is justified. We look at the disease statistically and understand that it is not familial and that the chance of its occurring twice in a small number of people is extremely remote. However, as a medical clerk, resident, or practicing physician, you will find that availability plagues you all the time, just as it plagues your patients. After you diagnose your first case of glioblastoma multiforme, you are likely to overreact to your next group of patients who complain of headaches. For the same reasons, you must be especially sensitive to the anxieties of the dizzy patient whose sister has multiple sclerosis, or of the mother of a child with vomiting and recent varicella infection whose nephew had Reye's syndrome.

You can avoid creating anxiety by being clear about why you need the information, sensitive to the patient's responses, and informative in your explanations.

- Make it clear that taking a family history is a routine part of your complete medical interview.

- Listen carefully for any emotional overlay or any connections made by the patient between family illnesses and his or her own.

- Demand no more detail than is required for your care of the patient.

- If the patient does become anxious, direct your attention to the anxiety by allowing the patient to express his or her concerns directly. In some cases, you may have to give an additive response (see Chap. 2) to relate the patient's free-floating anxiety to some unconsciously held causal belief (e.g., the coincidence of the patient's current age and her mother's age at the time she died).

S U M M A R Y : OAP, Past Medical History, Family History

In this chapter we discussed the importance of searching for other active medical problems (OAPs) in addition to the present illness:

- When you've completed the present illness, open the interview again with nondirective questions to search for OAPs.
- A question about current medications or other conditions under treatment is a good method of screening for OAPs.

The information you gather about the patient's past medical history helps to fill in the context of the present illness:

- Introduce the past medical history with a general question or statement, such as "I'd like to know a little more about how your health has been in the past."
- The level of detail you request about past illness should be dictated by present needs.
- Identify what the patient means by "allergy." Be sure to distinguish from side effects.

The family history is helpful for frankly mendelian diseases, family traits, and polygenetic conditions like heart disease, diabetes, and cancer:

- Be sensitive to the social dimension of the information you obtain, particularly in the family history.

References

1. Feinstein A. *Clinical Judgment*. Baltimore, Williams & Wilkins, 1967.
2. Eisenberg L, Kleinman A. Clinical social science. In: Eisenberg L, Kleinman A. (eds.) *The Relevance of Social Science for Medicine*. Dordrecht, Holland, D. Reidel, 1980.

Suggested Readings

Waters I, Watson W, Wetzel W. Genograms. Practical tools for family physicians. *Can Fam Physician* 1994; 40:282–287.

CHAPTER 5

Gaining Richness and Reality

• • •

THE PATIENT PROFILE

Dialogue . . . can exhibit the object from each point of view, and
show it to us in the round, as a sculptor shows us things,
gaining in this manner all the richness and reality of effect that
comes from those side issues that are suddenly suggested by
the central idea in progress, and really illumine the idea more
completely, or from those felicitous after-thoughts that give a
fuller completeness to the central scheme, and yet convey
something of the delicate charm of chance.

Oscar Wilde, *The Critic as Artist*

The patient profile, also called the **social history,** is the part of the medical
interview in which we attempt to learn something about the patient as a
person and how lifestyle influences his or her health. Illness is not simply
disordered pathophysiology; illness happens to a person and involves
changes in the person's feelings and abilities. Moreover, getting sick, seeking
care, getting well, and staying well all have social determinants. Patienthood
is a psychosocial role, not a biologic state, and knowledge of the patient as
a person is essential to the biopsychosocial approach to the patient. Thera-

peutic decisions involve not only medical judgments but also emotional, social, ethical, and interpersonal considerations.

The importance of the social history may not be readily apparent in the acute hospital setting, where the diagnostic and therapeutic objectives are set on an hour-to-hour (if not minute-to-minute) basis. In this artificial setting, knowing what the illness is like for the patient or what the patient's lifestyle is like seems much less important than knowing about the disease process. Yet this artificial view becomes irrelevant when it is time to discharge the patient, and the home environment and family support system become critical. For example:

- How many stairs will the patient have to climb?
- Who will prepare the food?
- How will he or she juggle the complicated medication schedule?
- How much will the patient's employment allow changes in lifestyle necessitated by the illness?
- What about disorders that are clearly occupational, such as back injuries in a young mother or carpal tunnel syndrome in a heavy equipment operator?

Hospital length of stay is much shorter now than it was only a few years ago; patients leave the hospital earlier in their period of recovery than used to be the case. Thus, when discharged they tend to be sicker and require more support in the home environment. Moreover, most medical care is not in the hospital at all. Most clinicians care for patients in their offices, and they deal with chronic and recurrent conditions that interact continuously with the patient's life circumstances.

Traditionally, we place the patient profile in a separate section of the written case history as if the social history were a self-contained aspect of the interview, but this is an arbitrary separation for the sake of organization only. You are continually acquiring social information throughout the interview from "small talk," the patient's manner of dress and speech, and demographic information that may appear on the chart. Another important aspect of your interaction is assessing educational level and intelligence, both of which are critical to your ability to communicate successfully; much of this assessment is done automatically as you converse at your patient's level of comprehension and in a manner appropriate to his or her life experience.

WHAT GOES INTO THE PATIENT PROFILE?

Just as it is a mistake to believe that there is such a thing as a "complete" review of systems, it is also a mistake to believe that there is a "complete" patient profile. You have time constraints. How do you limit the inquiry so as to avoid a lengthy assessment? What is relevant in the limited time you have? What information must be obtained when the patient is first admitted to the hospital or on the first office visit, and what can be developed over the course of a hospital stay or a long-term relationship with the patient? Unless the situation is emergent, your goal is to learn enough, at least, to answer three questions:

How do the patient's personal characteristics or lifestyle

- Contribute to the etiology of this illness?
- Aggravate or limit the severity of illness?
- Interfere or help with getting well?

The connection of certain illnesses with a patient's lifestyle is obvious, such as the development of recurrent viral infections among child care workers. At times, the social history is critical to making the diagnosis (sexually transmitted diseases and personality disorders are excellent examples); at other times, keeping the patient well depends on such factors as his or her ability to follow a special diet or a complex medical regimen.

A good way to begin the patient profile is with general questions such as:

- "Can you tell me a little about yourself? Your family? Your work?"
- "How have things been going for you otherwise? At home? At work? In your marriage?"

Often one of the most useful parts of an entire history is a detailed description of what the patient usually does on an ordinary day and exactly how this is modified by the illness. For example, in the case of a person who may be suffering from dementia, the description of a typical day may be more revealing than mental status testing, particularly when the dementia is mild. The description may be more clinically important as well, since what really counts is how the patient functions in his or her environment, not on a mental status test.

The degree of completeness that you need depends on the situation. Some information may emerge in the course of the interview without specific questioning; often data are acquired not on the first day of hospitalization or during the first office visit but over time as you get to know the patient and understand what is relevant to his or her care. Keep in mind that the idea is to find out the patient's strengths and weaknesses and the nature of his or her support system, if any. How has this person coped with illness or other stress in the past? How does he or she keep distress within manageable limits? Remember that more intimate data are more easily and reliably obtained when you know the patient better, whether later in your initial history, later in the interview, later in the hospitalization, or years later in your relationship with the patient. Tailor what you need to know to the situation at hand.

DEMOGRAPHICS AND OCCUPATION

The patient's age, education, race or ethnic background, religion, and residence are among the most fundamental data about the person. These characteristics affect risk of various diseases, beliefs about the causes of illness, and the ability to participate in recommended therapy. Often this information is provided for you on the "front sheet" filled in by office or hospital personnel when the patient registers or is admitted.

Data about employment, school, or retirement are vital to understanding the patient and to building an understanding of the patient's support system. Are there financial problems related to the patient's job or lack of a job? Is the retired person actively involved in hobbies or volunteer work? How does the patient cope with being a working wife and mother? How does the patient unwind from the rigors of daily living?

There are three essential points to a quick occupational survey that should be included in any medical history:

- Inquire about the patient's occupation and construct a short list of jobs he or she has held, particularly those held for a long time.
- Include one key screening question about exposure: "Do you now (or did you sometime in the past) have exposure to fumes, chemicals, dusts, loud noise, or radiation?"
- Explore any temporal relationship of the current medical problem to activities at work or at home, including job-related stress.

The key details are what the person actually does on the job. For example, a patient who "works for the phone company" may be a manager, a telephone installer, or a maintenance person who works out-of-doors on telephone lines. Similarly, a steelworker may operate heavy equipment, drive a truck, or work in an office. Each job exposes the patient to different risks, ranging from chronic stress to serious accidents. By not considering occupational exposures, clinicians miss the opportunity to diagnose certain acute and chronic illnesses. Table 5–1 presents various examples of occupational and environmental causes of medical problems.

CULTURAL AND HEALTH BELIEFS

Illness may affect the patient in many ways—from the trivial to the profound. There are day-to-day problems, such as getting up and down steps for a patient whose surgery or illness limits her ability to do so in a house with its only bathroom on the second floor, or the widower who eats out and must limit his sodium intake. Illness produces hardships of a different sort when it takes away the patient's ability to earn a living or renders the aging spouse unable to care for his or her mate. Illnesses also have an emotional impact; a woman with a localized breast cancer and a man with an

TABLE 5–1 OCCUPATIONAL AND ENVIRONMENTAL CAUSES OF MEDICAL PROBLEMS

Condition	Industry/Occupation	Agent
Pulmonary tuberculosis	Physicians, medical personnel	*Mycobacterium tuberculosis*
Plague, tularemia, anthrax, rabies, and other infections	Farmers, ranchers, hunters, veterinarians, laboratory workers	Various infectious agents
Rubella	Medical personnel, intensive care personnel	Rubella virus
Hepatitis	Day-care center staff, orphanage staff, medical personnel	Hepatitis A virus, hepatitis B virus
Malignant neoplasm of nasal cavities	Woodworkers, cabinet makers, furniture makers	Hardwood dust
	Radium chemists and processors	Radium
	Nickel smelting and refining	Nickel
Malignant neoplasm of larynx	Asbestos industries and utilizers	Asbestos
Malignant neoplasm of trachea, bronchus, and lung	Asbestos industries and utilizers	Asbestos
	Topside coke oven workers	Coke oven emissions
	Uranium and fluorspar miners	Radon daughters
	Smelters, processors, users	Chromates, nickel, arsenic
	Mustard gas formulators	Mustard gas
	Ion exchange resin makers, chemists	Bis(chloromethyl)ether
Mesothelioma	Asbestos industries and utilizers	Asbestos
Malignant neoplasm of bone	Radium chemists and processors	Radium
Malignant neoplasm of scrotum	Automatic lathe operators, metalworkers	Mineral/cutting oils
	Coke oven workers, petroleum refiners	Soots and tars
Malignant neoplasm of bladder	Rubber and dye workers	Benzidine, naphthylamine, auramine, 4-nitrophenyl
Malignant neoplasm of kidney	Coke oven workers	Coke oven emissions
Acute lymphoid leukemia	Radiologists, rubber industry	Ionizing radiation
Acute myeloid leukemia	Occupations with exposure to benzene	Benzene
	Radiologists	Ionizing radiation
Erythroleukemia	Occupations with exposure to benzene	Benzene
Aplastic anemia	Explosives manufacturers	TNT
	Radiologists, radium chemists	Ionizing radiation

(Continued on next page)

TABLE 5–1 OCCUPATIONAL AND ENVIRONMENTAL CAUSES OF MEDICAL PROBLEMS (*Continued*)

Condition	Industry/Occupation	Agent
Agranulocytosis or neutropenia	Explosives and pesticide industries	Phosphorus
	Pesticides, pigments, pharmaceuticals	Inorganic arsenic
Toxic encephalitis	Battery, smelter, and foundry workers	Lead
Parkinson's disease (secondary)	Manganese processing, battery makers, welders	Manganese
Inflammatory and toxic neuropathy	Pesticides, pigments, pharmaceuticals	Arsenic and arsenic compounds
	Furniture refinishers, degreasing operations	Hexane
	Plastics, rayon industries	Methyl butyl ketone, copper disulfide, other solvents
	Explosives industry	TNT
	Battery, smelter, and foundry workers	Lead
	Dentists, chloralkali plants, battery makers	Mercury
	Plastics industry, paper manufacturing	Acrylamide
	Microwave and radar technicians	Microwaves
	Radiologists	Ionizing radiation
	Blacksmiths, glass blowers, bakers	Infrared radiation
	Moth repellant formulators, fumigators	Naphthalene
Extrinsic asthma	Jewelry, alloy, and catalyst makers	Platinum
	Polyurethane, adhesive, paint workers	Isocyanates
	Plastic, dye, insecticide makers	Phthalic anhydride
	Foam workers, latex makers, biologists	Formaldehyde
	Bakers	Flour
	Woodworkers, furniture makers	Red cedar and other wood dust
Pneumoconiosis of coal workers	Coal miners	Coal dust
Asbestosis	Asbestos industries and utilizers	Asbestos
Silicosis	Quarrymen, sandblasters, silica processors, mining, ceramic industries, and foundries	Silica
Talcosis	Talc processors	Talc

TABLE 5–1 OCCUPATIONAL AND ENVIRONMENTAL CAUSES OF MEDICAL PROBLEMS
(*Continued*)

Condition	Industry/Occupation	Agent
Chronic beryllium disease of the lung	Beryllium alloy workers, ceramic and cathode ray tube makers, nuclear reactor workers	Beryllium
Byssinosis	Cotton industry workers	Cotton, flax, hemp, and cotton-synthetic dusts
Acute bronchitis, pneumonitis and pulmonary edema due to fumes and vapors	Alkali and bleach industries	
		Chlorine
	Silo fillers, arc welders	Nitrogen oxides
	Paper, refrigeration, oil industries	Sulfur dioxide
	Plastics industry	Trimellitic anhydride
Toxic hepatitis	Solvent utilizers, dry cleaners, plastics industry	Carbon tetrachloride, chloroform, trichloroethylene
	Explosives and dye industries	Phosphorus, TNT
	Fumigators, fire extinguisher formulators	Ethylene dibromide
Acute or chronic renal failure	Battery makers, plumbers, solderers	Inorganic lead
	Electrolytic processes, smelting	Arsine
	Battery makers, jewelers, dentists	Inorganic mercury
	Fire extinguisher makers	Carbon tetrachloride
	Antifreeze manufacturers	Ethylene glycol
Contact and allergic dermatitis	Leather tanning, poultry dressing plants, packing, adhesives and sealant industry, boat building and repair	Irritants (e.g., cutting fish oils, solvents, acids, alkalis, allergens)

SOURCE: Abbreviated and adapted from Landrigan PJ and Baker DB,[1] p. 600.

uncomplicated acute myocardial infarction may well have the same good prognosis, but in our society, a diagnosis of cancer is usually more devastating than a diagnosis of heart disease. For some, illness may have some positive consequences, such as for the person who believes physical suffering leads to spiritual enlightenment. For others, though, illness may represent a concrete sign of their failure to pray correctly or to have sufficient faith in God to be "healed." We consider sociocultural aspects of illness and the impact of the patient's health beliefs and expectations in Chapter 14.

LIFESTYLE

Nutrition and Diet

Detailed, practical information about nutrition may not be emphasized during your education. Your patients, on the other hand, may have strong beliefs about the role of diet in their health and illnesses. Many will have tried popular weight reduction plans and vitamin supplements. As a practitioner, you will be recommending dietary changes, such as reduction in fat intake fats or increase in dietary fiber, for both primary prevention and treatment of disease. If you have no idea about the person's basic eating habits, you will be unable to give appropriate advice. Specific food intolerance (e.g., lactose intolerance), food allergies, the condition of the patient's teeth, the ability to shop and prepare food, and income all affect dietary habits. Ethnic and cultural influences may be very resistant to change.

You should determine how many meals per day the person usually eats and roughly at what time, including what sort of snacks he or she likes. For example, you will encounter obese patients who tell you truthfully that they eat only one meal per day. They attempt to cut down and lose weight, but are continually frustrated in their efforts. "I hardly eat anything, yet everything I eat turns to fat . . . I just can't lose a pound." This problem may arise in part from their one-meal-per-day habit, which promotes frequent (sometimes continual) snacking during the rest of the day. This snacking may be an almost unconscious background phenomenon that the person fails to count as a meal.

Another aspect of dietary history is a picture of dietary composition, particularly with regard to fats, salt, fiber, and other food groups. Find out, for example:

- The proportion of red meat, compared with poultry or fish
- Percentage of fat, especially saturated fat (butter, dairy products, and cooking oils)
- Some indication of indigestible fiber intake (grains and leafy vegetables)
- How much salt cooked in or added to food ("Do you add salt when you cook or at the table?")

Perhaps the most accurate and efficient way to assess the patient's dietary habits is to ask, "Tell me what you've eaten over the last 24 hours beginning with just before you came to the office (for outpatients) and working back." And then, "Is this a typical day for you, or how is it different?" **The question "Tell me about your diet" may be misinterpreted if the patient is not on a weight-reduction diet.** Details are important. If the patient has toast for breakfast and a sandwich for lunch, find out what goes on the toast and between the two slices of bread.

Consideration also should be given to caffeine intake. It is not uncommon to find patients who routinely drink several cups of coffee per day, in addition to frequent cola beverages, and who increase this intake during periods of stress. Caffeine usage may help explain symptoms such as headaches, irritability, palpitations, fatigue, and lightheadedness.

Daily Activities and Exercise

Knowledge of the patient's demographic characteristics and occupation will give you some clues to the patient's lifestyle. How he or she spends a typical day reveals even more about factors that may contribute to illness or facilitate getting well. For example, the sedentary retired salesman will need an explicit and graded exercise program with frequent monitoring of his progress as he recuperates from a heart attack. People who are constantly on the go, eating on the run, and rarely preparing their own food may need to undertake major and difficult changes in lifestyle in order to treat obesity and hyperlipidemia.

Exercise is a major feature in the patient profile. Vague answers such as "I like to play tennis" or "I have a rowing machine at home" are not necessarily indicators of regular aerobic exercise. Perhaps the patient has not had time for tennis since the summer of 1991 or the rowing machine has sat unused for years in the basement. To monitor health effects, you must inquire specifically about regularity and duration, as well as manner, of exercise. As you do this, you can also assess the potential for various types of trauma that result from sports and exercise programs (e.g., stress fractures in joggers, major knee injuries in skiers).

Smoking, Alcohol, and Recreational Drugs

You should ascertain the amount, frequency, and context of these behaviors. Assessing truthfulness is a common problem when eliciting smoking, drug, and alcohol histories because these are loaded topics, and most people (both patients and physicians) feel that there are "right" and "wrong" answers to questions about them. For example, when asked "How much do you smoke?" many smokers reply "Too much." Notice how there is no quantification in this answer; the reply is colored by the patient's awareness that it is "wrong" to smoke. It may be easier for such patients to talk more neutrally about what age they started to smoke or how many times they have tried to quit.

Here is a smoking history obtained from a 40-year-old man presenting with shortness of breath. The physician tries to find out exactly how much is "not too much" and also tries to determine whether the patient's current respiratory symptoms caused him to cut down and whether the cumulative smoking history is sufficient to cause medical problems, like chronic bronchitis or perhaps carcinoma of the lung:

Dr: Okay. How much do you smoke?

Pt: Oh, not too much.

Dr: How much is not too much?

Pt: Oh, umm, not half a pack a day.

Dr: Is that as much as you've always smoked? Have you ever smoked more than that?

Pt: Uh, when I was barbering, I would smoke more, sometimes a pack. You know, but they would burn out. You know, because when I was doing a customer or something, they'd burn out, so I'd just light up another one.

Dr: Uh hmm. How old were you when you started?

Pt: Thirteen.

Similarly, use of drugs or alcohol is seen by most patients as a habit of which the physician will disapprove. Some will deny the use of these substances, particularly if asked a yes/no question. Here is an example of a physician (who can smell alcohol on the patient's breath) trying to elicit the history of alcohol use in a 28-year-old woman presenting for evaluation of hypertension:

Dr: . . . You are using some aspirin and Tylenol?

Pt: Every once in a while. It's not regular, but that's the only drugs I take.

Dr: And are you a pretty steady drinker?

Pt: I have one or two drinks at work, you know. After work I . . .

Dr: . . . Okay. Do you have any more than that?

Pt: Sometimes it's more than that but basically . . .

Dr: Is that something that would be hard for you to give up?

Pt: Well, it's a very social type thing for me, I guess . . . so . . . yeah, I'd have to think about it, ha ha.

Often in this situation it is not so much what the patient says, but how she says it. This patient paused and looked away, and began to use phrases such as "you know" and hedges like "basically." She also displayed some nervous laughter. These are often clues that a person is telling less than the truth. You may notice pauses (time to censor material), shifts in position, eye aversion, and hedges in the verbalization, such as "not really" instead of "no." The most revealing question in this example is the indirect one ("Is that something that would be hard for you to give up?"), to which the patient's answer ranges from denial ("Well, it's a very social type thing . . .") to agreement ("I guess so, yeah . . .") to ambivalence ("I'd have to think about it"). It is rarely useful to tell the patient that you doubt the accuracy of his or her story, especially when you have not already built a relationship. You should, however, make a mental note of the behavior in the hope that some time in the future you will be able to use the information to help the patient.

Another patient with a history of narcotic addiction, when asked about his current drug use, replied, "No, not much. I mean some. Yeah, I'm using." Illicit drug use and narcotic addiction, particularly when the physician is potentially the patient's source of drugs, is a difficult situation that demands careful attention to both the substance and style of the patient's statements.

RELATIONSHIPS

Support System

It is helpful to find out family composition—who lives with the patient (e.g., parents, grandparents, siblings, spouse, or children) and what their ages are. Widowed persons face special problems in coping with stress and, indeed, have higher rates of illness and death, particularly during the first year of widowhood. As you get to know the patient better, you can begin to discuss the stresses and satisfactions related to his or her family's functioning. You have begun to develop an idea of the patient's support system when you know the answers to questions such as the following:

- Are there family members nearby who are willing and able to help in time of crisis?
- What kind of help does the young mother have with her new baby?
- Who will care for the elderly, demented patient when her husband (who normally cares for her) has his hernia surgery?

For patients with chronic illness or disability, especially when there is no family or the family has limited financial or emotional resources, part of the clinician's role is to arrange for needed health services (e.g., transportation to the physician's office, home care, Meals-on-Wheels), usually with the help of social agencies.

Marital And Other Significant Relationships

As you begin to understand the patient's lifestyle, you also develop a sense of the patient's relationship with his or her spouse or significant other. You may not need to ask direct questions about this. Because patients may regard this information as intimate and possibly unrelated to their illness, it is best to ask questions in a somewhat indirect and open-ended manner, which permits patients to reveal as much or as little as they wish. You may begin, for example, with questions relating the patient's illness to the current state of the relationship: "How has doing (chronic peritoneal) dialysis affected your husband?" Such questions allow the patient to say anything from "Okay" to "Well, we've had our rough spots but things are pretty good right now" to "To tell you the truth, I keep wanting to leave him, but I can't." More specific questions, such as those that follow, are useful once the patient has indicated an interest in discussing the relationship:

- "What are some of the good and bad things about your present relationship?"
- "What would you change?"

In addition to the impact of illness on relationships and of relationships on illness, certain diagnoses or clues to diagnoses reside in the story of the patient's relationships. For example, the criteria for diagnosing certain personality disorders lie in the patient's history of difficult relationships with family, friends, and employers.

Domestic violence, long considered a strictly "private" matter by both health professionals and law enforcement alike, is now recognized as a serious public health problem, sufficiently prevalent to justify screening in the medical setting. Detecting relationships that are physically or emotionally abusive is an important function of the patient profile. Table 5–2 outlines an approach to screening for domestic violence that begins with less threatening and somewhat general questions, and progresses to more specific queries that focus on the patient's safety.[2,3] Note how each question allows the

---

TABLE 5–2 DETECTING DOMESTIC VIOLENCE: THE "SAFE" QUESTIONS

Stress/Safety
What stress do you experience in your relationships?
Do you feel safe in your relationships?
Should I be concerned for your safety?

Afraid/Abused
Are there situations in your relationships where you have felt afraid?
Has your partner ever threatened or abused you or your children?
Have you been physically hurt or threatened by your partner?
Has your partner forced you to have sexual intercourse that you did not want?

Friends/Family
If you have been hurt, are your friends or family aware of it?
Do you think you could tell them if it did happen?
Would they be able to give you support?

Emergency Plan
Do you have a safe place to go and the resources you need in an emergency situation?
If you are in danger now, would you like help in locating a shelter?
Would you like to talk with a social worker (a counselor, me) to develop an emergency plan?

SOURCE: Adapted from Ashur[2] and Neufeld.[3]

patient to answer from her point of view, avoiding judgmental wording and remaining open-ended.

SEXUAL HISTORY

Sexual functioning is an essential part of most patients' life experience and may be an important factor in illness. Depression, anxiety, and anger may relate to underlying sexual problems; conversely, many physical illnesses or diseases can lead to sexual dysfunction. Asking even a few questions about sexual functioning sends the message that the physician is willing to discuss sexual concerns if the patient wishes.

There is no requirement to get a complete sexual history from every patient. Sometimes one question ("Are you having any sexual problems?") suffices, and this question may be asked as part of the review of systems. If the patient answers in the negative, no more need be said; you have, however, indicated that sexual concerns are legitimate fare for discussion, to which the patient may return later if he or she wishes. Sometimes the patient's constellation of symptoms leads you to inquire more thoroughly about sexual behavior and functioning.

The patient may not expect a discussion of sexual matters, especially if he or she feels that the presenting complaint is unrelated to sex, or is accustomed to physicians who never ask about sexual functioning. For example, the young man presenting with severe sore throat may be very surprised at your interest in his sexual activity, unless you explain that his clinical syndrome and negative tests raise the possibility of gonococcal pharyngitis.

Knowing something about the patient as a person facilitates asking difficult questions about sexuality. For example, once you know whether the patient is married or is living with someone, it is easier to ask about sexual preference and activity. When in doubt, you should use the term "partner" rather than gender-specific terms such as "boyfriend" or "wife." If you ask only about opposite-sex partners, the patient may infer that you would be shocked by a report of gay or lesbian activity. The homosexual patient may, therefore, avoid relating his or her actual sexual preference. On the other hand, the happily married 65-year-old may well be offended by the use of the term "partner."

Delaying this part of the history until later in the interview will also allow you to become familiar with the patient's language and make it easier to use words that he or she can understand. As with other intimate bodily functions (voiding and defecating), patients may describe their sexual functioning with words conditioned by their age, level of education, and cultural background. Other descriptions may be idiosyncratic and obscure. What do words like "relationship," "birth control," or "safe sex" mean? Open-ended questions permit the patient to use his or her own words. In your follow-up questions, you then can use the patient's own words, thereby ensuring a common basis for understanding.

The sexual history can also be included in a nonthreatening way as part of the review of systems, for example, while dealing with gynecologic symptoms in women, or with genitourinary symptoms in men. The focus is always on the patient's own perception of whether there is a sexual problem, not a voyeuristic account of frequency or techniques. You should not probe if the patient does not wish to discuss the matter. You may continue with questions about other aspects of the health history, at the same time building rapport, and return to the sexual history, if necessary, when more trust exists.

Here are some examples of useful ways to initiate a discussion of sexuality:

- "Are you having any sexual problems?"
- "Do you have any questions or concerns about sexuality or sexual functioning?"
- "Many people who are ill experience a change in their sexual function. Have you noticed any change?"
- "Has your interest in sex changed recently? Since you've been ill?"
- "A lot of men have sexual problems when they take blood pressure medicine. Have you noticed any problems?"
- "It sounds as though your marriage has been a good one. How about your sexual relationship?"
- "Many girls (boys) your age have questions about sex and birth control. How about you?"
- "Many people these days worry about AIDS. Do you have any concerns about being at risk for AIDS?"

If the patient indicates problem areas, then proceed with more detailed questioning. Sexual dysfunction may result from any combination of physical, pharmacological, or emotional problems; explore the medical reasons that may account for or contribute to dysfunction and assess the emotional component. The history should be more extensive, for example, when a patient requests birth control, fears a sexually transmitted disease, or has a sexual problem as a presenting complaint. Consider this example of a patient whose chief complaint is pain during intercourse:

Dr: You don't look as tired as you were before.

Pt: I'm not as tired since I've been taking the iron pills.

Dr: That's helped, huh. Well, do you have another problem?

Pt: Yeah, with my stomach. When I have sex, my stomach hurts right here. After, that, it doesn't bother me.

Dr: When you have sex? Otherwise you feel good?

Pt: Uh huh.

Dr: Okay. When did all this start?

Pt: About a month ago.

Dr: And has it gotten any better since that time?

Pt: Uh uh, it's the same.

Dr: Has it gotten any worse?

Pt: Sometimes it gets worse.

Dr: When you're not having sex you feel fine?

Pt: Uh huh. But sometimes, when I walk, I get this real sore pain and then I get real bad.

Dr: When you have the pain during intercourse, is it all the time during intercourse or at the beginning or at the end? Or only when he is thrusting inside?

Pt: Right here.

Dr: Only on that side. Does it hurt anywhere else?

Pt: Uh uh.

Dr: Have you ever had this problem before?

Pt: It always did that.

Dr: So you've had this a long time.

Pt: Ah ha.

Dr: What made you think now it might be serious, even though it didn't get worse.

Pt: It gets worse sometimes. But I just get . . . but I just thought it was nothing.

Dr: Can you think of any reason why you want to get it checked now?

Pain on intercourse can be a sign of pelvic abnormality (pelvic inflammatory disease or endometriosis), underlying depression, or problems in the particular relationship. The physician in this example asks an open-ended question ("Do you have another problem?") and then Wh questions ("When did all this start?" "Does it hurt anywhere else?" "Can you think of any reason why you want to get it checked now?"). The physician also uses more specific questions to obtain precise details ("When you have the pain during intercourse, is it all the time during intercourse or at the beginning or at the end? Or only when he is thrusting inside?"). Because many patients have difficulty discussing such details, the physician gives her a number of choices from which to choose her answer. This reticent patient, however, avoids answering entirely and, instead, points to the location of her pain. The physician obtains the useful information that the pain is limited to one side but still does not know at what part of intercourse it occurs.

In this example, it would be helpful to know if the patient's desire—libido—has changed ("Do you feel like making love—having sex—as much as you used to?") or if her ability to enjoy sex has changed ("Do you feel satisfied when you make love?"). Choose words that the patient can understand. If you are not sure you are being understood, ask ("Do you understand what I am asking?"). As much as possible, you should ask questions that permit patients to answer from their own point of view and in their own way (e.g., "Do you feel satisfied?" as opposed to "Do you have an orgasm?").

When you suspect a sexually transmitted disease, it will be necessary to know about sexual preference, as well as number and regularity of sexual partners, and to ask if the partners have had any sexually transmitted disease symptoms. These are difficult topics because a sexually transmitted disease may be embarrassing for the patient, and he or she may not want to acknowledge that a partner may have gone outside the relationship. Patients may feel anger and guilt or may perceive the physician as accusatory.

You should express your questions in the same neutral way that you talk about other illnesses or infections: "Are you concerned that you might have gotten this from someone?" or "Is there any chance that you have been exposed to someone with a similar infection?" Sometimes it helps to introduce a difficult question with a statement, such as "I think you may have an infection that is acquired only during sexual intercourse, but I don't want to make any assumptions about your sexual relationships. Is it possible that you've been with someone who has the same thing?" If the patient says "That's impossible," accept that statement as representing the patient's belief. You can still add, "If you do think of anybody who might have this, it would be good if you could tell them to get checked." Do not argue with the patient. If the diagnosis is uncertain, say so and outline the plan for making the diagnosis clear. In the case of reportable venereal diseases, the clinician might say, "By law, I am required to report this illness, and there may be someone from the health department who will talk to you about who else might have it."

Another difficult situation arises with teenagers (see Chapter 8). Sexually active teenagers are, of course, at risk for sexually transmitted disease and pregnancy. In evaluating any genitourinary or pelvic problem, it is therefore necessary to ask about sexual activity. Some 13-year-old girls have been pregnant, while others have little knowledge of sexuality at all. It is helpful to begin with the patient's interest in school, social activities, then "boys" or "girls," and finally sex. Some helpful questions are:

- "Do you have any questions about your body? About sex? About how not to get pregnant?"
- "Are your friends or the kids at school into having sex yet? How about you?"
- "Some girls (boys) your age get pretty serious about boys (girls) and start having sex. How about you?"

Patients should be allowed to answer in their own way, with your assurance that the information will be confidential. Men should be questioned about their risk of getting someone pregnant, just as much as women should be asked about their risk of pregnancy.

Here is an example of the kind of sexual problem that arises frequently in medical patients. You should determine if the problem is the result of medication side effects, difficulties in the relationship, or some combination of factors.

Dr: . . . Are you living at home now? Living with your boyfriend?

Pt: He's like 16 years older than me and we've been together for about 15 years, but see there's a, a little bit of a problem when we have to, 'cause see since I've been on those steroids, you know it messes with your sex life, too. I don't have any.

Dr: You don't have any desire?

Pt: No, and uh, that creates a problem. I just have no desire. It was like if he put his hands on me, I might get real evil, you know, like "get your hands off of me," you know.

Dr: I see. How are things between you and him otherwise? Are things strained in general?

Pt: I wish he would get out of my life.

One final note: Many people also want to know what is "normal" in sexual matters and discern whether they fit the normal standard. They may ask your opinion. Do not confuse being genuine with giving personal details of your own life. Some questions that patients may put to you are clearly inappropriate ("What would you do? Would you have an abortion?" or "Did you have sex before you got married?"), and it is best to answer in a polite and straightforward manner, "Well, we're not here to discuss what I think. I'm more interested in finding out how you feel about this pregnancy (or about learning that your daughter is gay)." In this way, you will help the patient explore his or her own feelings and symptoms as opposed to yours, which are not the focus of the interview.

THE PATIENT PROFILE AT WORK

Here are several examples that demonstrate the importance of the social history or patient profile in the diagnosis and management of medical problems. In the first example, a 61-year-old African-American woman with diabetes and hypertension urgently scheduled a visit to her family physician, complaining of chest pain, headache, and increasing concern about her blood pressure. The physician, confused about which problem was really the chief complaint (since the symptoms were chronic and the blood pressure under control), asked the patient to clarify her concerns:

Dr: Uh, what, what would you say is the thing that's worrying you the most right now?

Pt: Well, mostly, is how, getting those bills paid. See, I'm on, I'm on assistance.

Dr: Oh, I see. Tell me more about this worry. Did something new happen?

Pt: Mostly it's a gas bill and then, um, see I own a house. I have the taxes, keeping up with them, and, ah, just finances generally.

Dr: Did you recently get your gas bill?

Pt: Yes, I did.

Dr: When did that come?

Pt: Yes, ah, it came the other day.

In this instance, the social problem was **the** problem. Notice how the physician looked for positive or confirmatory evidence that it was her inability to pay the gas bill that was really bothering the patient. This doesn't mean that her chest pain, headaches, and high blood pressure weren't "real," but it was very helpful in answering the "why now" question—that is, why the patient sought care at this particular time for symptoms that had not changed.

Next, consider an example in which another social determinant of the decision to seek care becomes apparent:

Pt: See, um, I used to, okay, I used to do hair, I'm a barber, I'd do a lotta hair, so I had to go to, uh, um, I had to go to the clinic. Okay, now barbers every time they get their license renewed, they have to go to the health department.

Dr: Right.

Pt: Right. Okay and they gave, uh, they gave me some pills to take because they gave me a test, um, humm, and it came back positive . . .

Dr: Um humm.

Pt: You know they gave me some pills to take, they say I have to take them for a year.

Dr: Um humm.

Pt: But before the end of the year, after I run out, I'm supposed to come back and get some more . . .

Dr: Right, I see . . .

Pt: And I didn't.

Here, a patient with chest pain is probably concerned that his failure to follow up on recommended treatment for a positive tuberculin test may be the etiology of his current symptoms. The only reason he had the tuberculin test in the first place was to satisfy the state licensing requirements to be a barber.

The final example is a patient in whom a variety of lifestyle factors contribute to his illnesses, which include obesity, headaches, and secondary syphilis:

Pt: The thing that is interesting to me is I am busy and I am constantly on my feet and I must put in at least 4 miles each day, but it doesn't affect my weight because of the types of things I eat. I don't eat heavily, it's just the things I eat.

Dr: How do you mean?

Pt: When I have not eaten for a whole day, I go to some deli and grab a creampuff and go to bed. That gives me sugar, and sugar helps me. Sugar really helps me keep elevated. I have a terrible—well, I have to drink orange drink. I don't eat breakfast, as a matter of fact, I only eat one meal a day, but it's a junk meal. And I'm very hooked on, I have to have a sugar-type drink in the morning to get elevated. Could use one now!

Dr: Now that you know all these things, is there any way you can change something? Like when you go to New York, you can find some time for yourself, even if it's sitting down for 10 minutes, instead of 10 seconds?

Pt: I lived there for 2 years, and when I started the business, I didn't realize at the time that the business was going to grow as quickly as it did, and I found out I was going to New York more and staying in hotels. Hotel living is disgusting. All I want to do is—my day starts at usually 6:30 or 7:00 o'clock in the morning and sometimes ends at 10:00 or 11:00 at night. And all I want to do is go back to the hotel, shove some sugar in my face, and go to sleep. This is the part where it gets into the personal part of it. My lifestyle changed quite a bit; a lot of things changed for me. I have always felt that I had very strong religious convictions and things like that. When I moved to New York, my lifestyle totally changed. I had to be very social; I wasn't a very social person. I wasn't a party person, I wasn't a drug person. But I went to parties where everybody was having sex with everybody else and you really didn't even get to know the person. You may never see them again and that type of thing. Well, all these things happened to me in this period. And I have to be honest with you, they frightened me, but I enjoyed them. I knew they were wrong, but there was a part of me that enjoyed them. So I was getting very confused. I felt that it was time for me to come back.

Dr: You felt that this was a way of coming back home?

> **Pt:** Exactly. What happened to me recently was that because of me going back to the way I wanted to be and things not working out the way I thought they should, so I figured why should I make sacrifices and be this person. You know, and not getting the results I want from it. I'll go back to being the other person. And I went back to being the other person and I got (laughing loudly) a social disease! Now you know my life story. That's it in a nutshell.

Note how the physician skillfully uses open-ended questions ("How do you mean?") and interchangeable responses ("You felt this was a way of coming back home?")

This patient (whom we met briefly in Chapter 1) acquired syphilis, probably at a party at which he had multiple sexual partners. He was finding his obesity difficult to control and was experiencing constant fatigue and stress-related tension (muscle contraction) headaches. His syphilis, which had advanced to the secondary stage with the development of a rash before it was diagnosed, became public evidence of what the patient saw as religious transgressions. He was dreadfully afraid that he had been exposed to HIV during his semianonymous gay sex. His anxiety and guilt made it difficult for him to work as hard as he felt he needed to in order to keep his business going. This patient did, indeed, develop AIDS and died about 2 years later.

S U M M A R Y : The Patient Profile

We close this chapter with a table (Table 5–3) displaying key elements of the patient profile and some typical questions you might ask to begin to explore these elements. These questions are by no means a screening algorithm; they are simply examples of how one might choose to screen for these elements on an initial visit with the patient.

TABLE 5–3 ELEMENTS OF THE PATIENT PROFILE

Topics	Typical Screening Questions
Demographics and Occupation Age, gender, race, ethnic group, religion, marital status, education, occupation	Now that I know something about your symptoms, tell me a little about yourself. All I know is that you're 53 years old and married. What kind of work do you do? What exactly does that job involve?

TABLE 5–3 ELEMENTS OF THE PATIENT PROFILE (*Continued*)

Topics	Typical Screening Questions
Health Beliefs and Expectations (see Chap. 14)	What are you hoping to get out of this visit today?
	Do you have any concerns about taking medication?
Lifestyle	
Nutrition and diet	What's your diet like? Tell me what you eat on an average day.
Daily activities and exercise	
Cigarette, alcohol, and drug use	Tell me a bit about yourself.
	What is an average day like for you?
	Do you have time for regular exercise?
	Any concerns over your use of alcohol? Do you smoke cigarettes?
Relationships	
Family and household composition	Now tell me about your family. You've been married how long? Children?
Support system	
Marital and other significant relationships	Any stresses or problems with your family?
Sexual history	Any problems in your marriage?

References

1. Landrigan PJ, Baker DB. The recognition and control of occupational disease. *JAMA* 1991; 266:676–680.
2. Ashur ML. Asking about domestic violence: SAFE questions [letter]. *JAMA* 1993; 269:2367.
3. Neufeld B. SAFE questions: Overcoming barriers to the detection of domestic violence. *Am Fam Physician* 1996; 53:2575–2580.

Suggested Reading

Newman LS. Occupational illness. *N Engl J Med* 1995;333:1128–1134.

Shapiro J, Lenahan P. Family medicine in a culturally diverse world: A solution-oriented approach to common cross-cultural problems in medical encounters. *Fam Med* 1996; 28:249–255.

Wedding D (ed). *Behavior and Medicine*. St. Louis, Mosby–Year Book, 1995.

CHAPTER 6

No Air of Finished Knowledge

• • •

REVIEW OF SYSTEMS, PHYSICAL EXAMINATION, AND CLOSURE

A physician of this kind never gives a servant any account of his complaint, nor asks him for any; he gives him some empirical injunction with an air of finished knowledge in the brusque fashion of a dictator, and then is off in hot haste to the next ailing servant . . .

Plato, *The Laws*

THE REVIEW OF SYSTEMS

The **review of systems** (ROS) demonstrates your responsibility for the total patient and may uncover significant symptoms or problems not otherwise elicited. Clinicians who feel uncertain about how to conduct an interview, or about their ability to integrate data, sometimes take refuge in a long, detailed ROS. They ask in great detail about every possible symptom, as if it were possible to get all the information simply by asking a comprehensive set of questions. Alternatively, other physicians look upon the ROS as a pro forma detail of little value—in other words, a burden.

What, then, are the goals of the ROS? First, to uncover any additional active medical problems not yet discussed; and, second, to identify additional symptoms that may be related to, or influence, the symptoms for which the patient is seeking help. The physician may ask questions to address these ends at any time during the interview. The ROS as a specific segment may be "emptied" when the relevant information is obtained elsewhere.

Platt and McMath observed more than 300 clinical interviews conducted by medical residents and delineated five syndromes of "clinical hypocompetence."[1] They called one of the syndromes "flawed database" and illustrated it with this vignette:

> The clinical interview took 44 minutes to complete. Time allocation was as follows: introduction=1 minute; definition of chief complaint (cardinal symptom) and development of present illness=15 minutes; major past medical events, health hazards (smoking, alcohol, medications), and family illnesses=8 minutes; and review of systems=20 minutes.[1]

In this case, the interview was structured in such a way that its efficiency in generating data was very poor. A large portion was devoted to a review of systems; this is generally unnecessary when one uses earlier parts of the interview to develop an understanding of the patient's life, habits, interests, and other active medical problems, as well as a skillful exploration of the current illness. The authors point out that a more functional allocation of time might be:

- Introduction (1 min)
- Understanding the patient's life, habits, and interests (5 min)
- Definition of chief complaint and present illness (15 min)
- Definition of other active medical problems (5 min)
- Major past medical and family history (8 min)
- ROS (3 min)[1]

As you gain experience, much of the ROS may be conducted while you perform the physical examination. As you examine the patient's ears, you might ask if he or she has had any problems with hearing, ear infections, and so forth; as you examine the eyes, you might ask if he or she wears glasses. This method of doing an ROS, however, requires a high level of competence. An additional problem is that the patient may believe that you are asking your question (e.g., "Are you having any headaches?") because of something that you see during the physical examination. This may create anxiety and distort the patient's response. Thus, it is important to preface your examination, or at least your questions, with a comment that you will be asking routine questions for the sake of completeness rather than questions specifically related to the patient's illness or physical findings.

Some practicing physicians approach the ROS with a standardized questionnaire that the patient fills out prior to seeing the doctor (see Chap. 12). The use of such an instrument, however, does not replace an ROS section of the interview but merely changes its character. Instead of asking directly about symptoms, the physician reviews the questionnaire and asks for more detail regarding positive responses. The clinician also must determine that the patient has, indeed, understood the written words well enough to answer the questions accurately. A questionnaire is perfectly acceptable, but it is useful for the learner to conduct a complete ROS without the benefit of such instruments. Then, after you have developed a comfortable style, you might create a personalized questionnaire for future use. You must also check out **pertinent negatives**; that is, symptoms a patient has not reported that would, if he or she had them, support one of your diagnostic hypotheses. If a patient presents with cough, a pertinent negative might be a lack of shortness of breath.

Several guidelines are useful in learning about and conducting a good ROS.

- It is not necessary to ask detailed questions about every symptom related to every organ system. **You can expand the net of your inquiry by first emphasizing symptoms related to the patient's principal complaint and by starting with general as opposed to yes/no questions.** For example, you can ask, "Are you having any trouble with your vision?" rather than "Is your vision decreasing?" or "Do you see double?" In other words, ask the patient about general difficulties with each system, then focus in on details of existing symptoms, and finally check out pertinent negatives.

- The ROS should be abbreviated or eliminated in emergency situations; it also can be completed at a later date if the patient is too tired or too sick to respond to a tedious inquiry at present.

- Anyone, even someone in perfect health, is likely to have some positive responses on a complete ROS. With each positive response, you should obtain enough detail to indicate whether the symptom is significant or trivial. As a general rule, significance relates to severity and duration: the more severe and the more chronic the symptom, the more likely it is to be important.

- The use of ambiguous terms such as indigestion, bowel trouble, or fatigue is adequate for initial screening. Then, if there is a positive response, the symptom can be defined more precisely.

- The ROS section of the history should be at the end of the interview so that you have had time to "size up" the patient and ascertain how to assess his or her responses (e.g., denial on the one hand or obsession with the trivial on the other).

The following transcript provides an example ROS. It is neither comprehensive nor ideal, but simply a reasonable example conducted by a medical house officer. As you read through this interview, think about how you might have phrased these questions, whether you feel important information is missing, and whether you feel any questions are excessively detailed:

Dr: I'm going to ask you a bunch of questions I ask everybody. They are very general questions and some of them have short answers. Do you find that you get fevers often?

Pt: No.

Dr: How about chills? Have you had any chills recently?

Pt: Yes, but I just took that as being, you know my hormones for my hysterectomy. That's what I took it as being.

Dr: Okay. Do you get night sweats?

Pt: Yes.

Dr: Do you soak through all your bed clothing?

Pt: No.

Dr: How much do you weigh now?

Pt: 202.

Dr: How much did you weigh a year ago?

Pt: About 180–190.

Dr: What is the most you have ever weighed?

Pt: This.

Dr: You certainly aren't losing weight right now. Is that right?

Pt: Right.

Dr: Do you get headaches?

Pt: Sometimes. Maybe I'd say once a month. Maybe once every other month.

Dr: Do you have problems with your vision?

Pt: No.

Dr: Do you ever have double vision?

Pt: No.

Dr: Ever see spots in front of your eyes?

Pt: No.

Dr: How about blurry vision?

Pt: No.

Dr: Have you ever passed out?

Pt: No.

Dr: Blacked out?

Pt: No.

Dr: Do you often feel lightheaded?

Pt: No.

Dr: Do you hear ringing in your ears?

Pt: No.

Dr: Do you get a pain in your throat?

Pt: No.

Dr: Sore throats often?

Pt: No.

Dr: Does your neck hurt?

Pt: No.

Dr: Have you noticed any lumps or bumps anywhere in your body?

Pt: No.

Dr: Do your joints ache?

Pt: Yes.

Dr: Which ones?

Pt: Here.

Dr: Okay, you are pointing to your left knee and your back. How about other joints in your body?

Pt: No.

Dr: Do your muscles ache?

Pt: I just thought that it was my muscles in my leg.

Dr: Okay, fine. Do you get short of breath when you exercise?

Pt: I haven't exercised.

Dr: How about just walking around town?

Pt: No.

Dr: Can you climb stairs without becoming short of breath?

Pt: Yes.

Dr: Do you get pain in your chest?

Pt: No.

Dr: Have you ever gotten pain in your chest while you were exercising?

Pt: No.

Dr: Have you ever felt your heart fluttering or racing very quickly?

Pt: I don't think so.

Dr: Do your ankles swell on you?

Pt: No.

Dr: Are you able to lie flat in bed without becoming short of breath?

Pt: Yes.

Dr: Do you ever wake up in the middle of the night short of breath?

Pt: No.

Dr: Do you have to cough often?

Pt: No.

Dr: Ever cough up blood?

Pt: No.

Dr: Have you noticed any change in bowel habits, your bowel functions?

Pt: Yes.

Dr: How have they changed?

Pt: I don't pass my bowels as often as I did before I had surgery.

Dr: How often do you pass your bowels now?

Pt: Maybe twice a week.

Dr: Is the stool shaped as it was before or is it different? Is it thicker or thinner?

Pt: Thicker. Yeah, because a lot of times I have to chew some Feenamints to make it go myself.

Dr: Do you have diarrhea intermixed with this at all?

Pt: No.

Dr: Have you noticed any tarry black stools?

Pt: No.

Dr: How about blood in your stools or on your stools?

Pt: No.

Dr: Have you had any belly pain?

Pt: Yeah.

Dr: Where does your belly hurt you?

Pt: Right where I had my incision. Sometimes like only when I laugh.

Dr: It hurts you along the incision?

Pt: Uh-huh.

Dr: How about somewhere else in your belly?

Pt: Right here.

Dr: Okay, you are pointing to your right groin area.

Pt: It's just like—mostly like when I see something real funny and just like when I laugh. There is not any pain, it's just there. I just get a pain when I start laughing.

Dr: Have you noticed if you are very thirsty often? Do you find yourself drinking a lot of fluids?

Pt: Sometimes.

Dr: Do you think that you get cold more easily than some of your friends? Do you find that you put on heavy clothing when other people are not wearing jackets and things?

Pt: No.

Dr: Does the heat bother you more than you think it bothers other people?

Pt: No.

Dr: What is your energy level like?

Pt: So-so. It's moderate.

Dr: Do you become fatigued easily?

Pt: Sometimes.

Dr: How's your appetite?

Pt: Great.

What are the good and not-so-good features of this ROS? Among its good features are its completeness (almost every organ system is covered) and the way in which it is introduced. Also, the physician asks one question at a time and gives the patient sufficient opportunity to respond. However, there are also some problems. For example, the physician introduces a little medical jargon with the terms "night sweats" and "change in bowel habits," although many patients understand these terms. The more striking problem (and one common to the ROS) is the variation between lack of detail for some symptoms and overly elaborate detail for others. For example, the patient's complaints of headache, joint pains, and thirst are not further characterized; the clinician seems to have dismissed these symptoms as unimportant without additional inquiry. On the other hand, there appear to be too many specific questions on cough and various types of shortness of breath; one question, such as, "Do you have any trouble breathing?" would do.

The trick is to achieve balance. Because the physician is asking questions presumably unrelated to the main problem, the ROS serves as a screening device. The questions are not hypothesis-driven, and the probability that a positive response indicates significant pathology is low. Another way of putting this is that **the positive predictability (how often a certain symptom or symptom complex actually signifies a certain disease) of ROS responses is less than the positive predictability of spontaneous statements that arise in the course of the patient's elaboration of the present illness.**

The Positive ROS

Some patients give a very literal interpretation to the questions in an ROS, answering "yes" to almost every question. When this happens the task seems to be interminably tedious, and the interviewer fears that the history will never end. Sometimes, in addition to being positive, the answers are also given in great detail about relatively trivial matters. For example, while you may want to know if the patient wears glasses, you may have little interest in the fine details of how the patient's refractive error has changed in the past 5 years or what the patient feels about his or her optometrist. A difficult ROS might begin this way:

Dr: Now I'd like to ask you a series of questions just to make sure we haven't missed anything important, okay?

Pt: Fine.

Dr: I'll start with your head, and we'll work our way down. Do you get headaches?

Pt: Oh, I'm used to terrific headaches all through my life, and one doctor said it was high blood pressure, though I didn't know it at the time.

We seem to be off to a bad start as we do not expect or desire a severe, chronic problem to surface for the first time in the ROS; now, instead of zipping down the list of questions, the interviewer has to stop and ask the details about the headaches. When this happens, usually one of two things is going on: either the physician has failed to inquire in an empathic way about other active problems and significant past medical history, or the patient has simply over-interpreted the question.

The best way to deal with this situation is to prevent it by asking about other active problems and significant past medical problems soon after the questions concerning the present illness. Not only does this maneuver uncover such problems early in the interview but it also facilitates seeing connections between these problems and the present illness. If this technique fails or if you forget to use it, you might try one of a number of other approaches:

- Bring the patient back to the present with a reminder that the focus is on currently distressing symptoms.

- Make the questions very general – "Have you ever had any stomach or bowel trouble?"—and ask for further details only when the initial screening is positive.

- Encourage filtering out of unnecessary details by reminding the patient of time limitations, or by asking him or her to pick out the most important symptoms.

- Undertake the ROS while performing the physical examination and save time in that way.

TRANSITION TO THE PHYSICAL EXAMINATION

Medical interviewing, unlike other forms of the helper-client interaction, usually also involves a physical examination. The history and physical examination are different parts of the same process, a process that also includes negotiation, education, and clarification of plans. If we focus on data gathering, it is difficult to pinpoint exactly where the history ends and the physical examination begins, or vice versa. For example, from the first moment the patient walks into your office or you walk into the hospital room, you begin to make observations about the physical condition of the patient: You observe skin color, affect, behavior, and mental status. The entire mental status examination, although part of the interview in that it involves no touching, is really more properly considered as part of the systematic physical examination. On the other side of the coin, as you are doing the physical examination you continue to interact with your patient, hoping to obtain not only physical but also personal and symptom information.

It is difficult, at first, to go from talking to touching. Early in your medical experience, it is especially difficult to unglue yourself from your chair and approach the patient. In the hospital, paying attention to the patient's comfort, such as offering some water or changing the window blinds, may be appropriate. Ordinarily, when in the clinic or in your office, you will be interviewing a patient who is fully clothed. Although having a patient disrobe and put on an examination gown prior to the interview is often conducive to good office functioning, it is rarely conducive to patient comfort. It undermines respect for the person. Thus, the patient should be fully clothed, and you will be faced with telling him or her to get undressed when you are ready to start the examination. You should be quite direct and clear about what is going to happen and why.

- First, give the patient an opportunity for the last word. For example, "I think that's about it for now. Is there anything else we haven't covered or that you'd like to tell me before I examine you?"

- Second, tell the patient clearly what the game plan is. For example, "Next I'm going to do your physical examination, and then after that, we can sit down and talk about your problems and what tests you might need."

- Third, be very specific about what clothing the patient should remove, where he or she should sit or lie, and in what position. For example, "I'm going to step out of the room for a moment now. Please get undressed down to your underpants and put on this gown. Put it on with the opening toward the back. And then sit on the end of the table up here."

Here is how one physician begins an examination of a new patient. Note the explicit directions as well as the ROS-type question the physician asks at the beginning of the examination:

Dr: Do you have any questions before we do your exam?

Pt: No.

Dr: Okay. Why don't you climb up here, and just sit there, just step around, and come around there. Okay. I am going to cover you and you can just sit there. I'm going to check your thyroid and your lungs and your heart, and examine your breasts. Have you had any thyroid trouble?

Pt: No.

It is best for you to leave the room, or to pull a curtain across the room if one is available, while your patient gets undressed. In the hospital, of course, this is usually not a problem, but, even there, patients may want to use the bathroom or remove a dressing gown or robe. In office practice, when you are doing only part of a physical examination, it may be appropriate for the patient to remove only his or her shirt or unbutton several buttons. For specific parts of the examination, ask the patient to disrobe that area or, alternatively, say, "I'm going to untie (or unbutton or remove). . . ." If a female patient has large breasts, ask her for assistance in moving the breast in order for you to listen to the heart. This approach allows the patient to feel more like a participant and less like a victim.

CONVERSATION DURING THE PHYSICAL EXAMINATION

While maintaining a conversation during the physical examination allows you to continue to gather data, it may serve other essential functions as well. You can use your communication skills to put the patient at ease, encourage the patient to feel like an active participant in his or her own care, and diminish the perception of a difference in power between the physician and patient, which becomes more marked during the physical examination. Here is how one patient described it:

> Whether it be horizontal, or in some awkward placement on one's back or stomach, with legs splayed or cramped, or even in front of a desk, the patient is placed in a series of passive, dependent, and often humiliating positions. These are positions where embarrassment and anger are at war with the desire to take in what the doctor is saying. In this battle learning is clearly the loser.[2]

You also can use conversation to show the patient that you remember the complaint about abdominal pain while you are doing the abdominal examination, or you may use "small talk" to distract the patient so the patient's muscles will relax, making the abdominal or pelvic examination easier for the patient and more accurate as well.

Keep talking during the examination to gather further information, reassure the patient, and explain what you are doing. It may not be possible as a beginner to make comments while you also are concentrating on the sequence of things to do and the techniques for doing them. It is not difficult, however, to make such observations as:

- "I'm going to look into your ears now."
- "I'm feeling for your thyroid gland. Can you swallow now? I know it's difficult to swallow like that when someone asks you. Good."
- "I'm going to do a rectal exam now to check your prostate gland. It will make you feel like you are going to have a bowel movement, but don't worry, you won't."

It is also easy for you, and reassuring for the patient, to indicate that parts of your examination are normal. It is usually not particularly helpful to comment on every little thing you do, but if you know the patient is concerned about a particular system, it would be helpful to note your findings about that system right away. For the patient who comes in with chest pain, a comment that the heart and lungs sound normal can be quite reassuring for the patient (who need not be bothered at this point with the academic information that the heart may sound normal even when there is heart disease). Here is an example of how a physician spoke to a patient during the parts of the physical examination that involved listening to the lungs and heart and palpating the breasts and abdomen. Notice the insertion of a few ROS-type questions as the physician examines a part, education about self–breast examination, and attention to the patient's comfort ("Tell me if I hit any sore places."):

Dr: Okay, I am just going to loosen this (unties gown in back). How long have you been smoking?

Pt: About 3 years . . .

Dr: And you want to quit.

Pt: Well, yeah, I been thinking about it.

Dr: Take a deep breath. Okay, out, good, and again . . . Good. Now I am going to ask you to slip your arms all the way out and I am going to listen to your heart . . . Okay. Sounds good. Now I'm going to check your breasts. I want you to put your hands up like this (physician demonstrates) and I'm just going to look at them first to see if there are any bumps. . . .

Pt: Uh mm.

Dr: Okay, have you ever tried it?

Pt: No, not really.

Dr: We recommend that everyone do it once a month; the best time is right after your period has stopped. Do your breasts get sore before your period?

Pt: Yes.

Dr: Okay, well, that is why it is best to wait until after your period starts when usually the lumpiness goes away and they're not tender to touch. . . . I am going to ask you to just hold this up . . . and I want you to put your arms up over your head. What you do when you are checking is to do exactly what I'm doing. . . . Go all around the outside of your breasts like this . . . up here is breast tissue and also up here . . . so you are going to go in kind of a circle like this . . . then spiral in until you get every part including under the nipple. Okay? Now I'd like you to lie down and we'll check your breasts again. . . . We always check them in two positions. . . . And I am going to check your heart. . . . Do you have any indigestion or trouble with your bowels? Now tell me if I hit any sore places.

The pelvic examination is a particularly personal and anxiety-producing experience. You should explain clearly what you are about to do and what the patient is likely to feel. Ask the patient if she has had a pelvic examination before. Whether she has or not, it is very reassuring to say something like "I'm going to pretend that this is your first pelvic examination and explain everything that I'm doing." The less experience the patient has had, either with pelvic examinations or with you, the more reassurance she will need. You should first touch the patient's inner thigh and then firmly but gently conduct the examination. You should describe the anatomy to the patient as you are doing the examination. As you become more experienced, you will be able to help her relax her muscles through your calm tone of voice, your gentle palpation, and your instructions about deep, slow breathing.

Here is how one physician introduced a patient (who requested a diaphragm for birth control) to her first pelvic examination; everything is described with a relaxing, almost hypnotic, tone of voice, the physician's gestures are slow and deliberate (no sudden moves), and the physician continuously looks at the patient's face to gauge her reactions:

Dr: The next thing I am going to do is a pelvic exam. These are all the things I am going to use, but I am not going to use all of them on you. Okay. These are the slides on which the Pap test is done, and these are the swabs that I use to do the Pap test. They're just like long Q-tips, okay, and this also, which I will roll around the cervix just like that (demonstrating), see, it is not sharp. . . . We usually do a culture for infection at the same time. . . .

Pt: A culture?

Dr: Yes, and that is to check for infection. This instrument is cold, and that is really the worst thing about it. It is called a speculum and this is inserted very gently into the vagina and then opened very gently like that (demonstrating) so that I can see your cervix and see that it is normal. Okay? (Patient nods.)

Dr: What I will ask you to do is to put your feet into these things, which are called stirrups, these metal things, that's good, and now I want you to pull yourself all the way down to the end of the table like that, and practically feel yourself like your bottom is coming off the end of the table. Okay? That's fine. I am going to put this pillow under your head right there, okay, and I am going to shine a light on you so that I can see what I am doing and as I do things I will tell you what I am doing. Okay? Are you more or less comfortable?

Pt: I guess so.

Dr: All right, it is not very comfortable, that is true. Okay. Now what I am going to do is to look at the outside of you first. If you can just kind of relax, that's good. Now what I am doing is checking the labia, or lips. Good. Now you are going to feel my finger at the edge of the vagina, feeling where your cervix is. Do you know what your cervix is?

Pt: No.

Dr: Okay, that is the opening to your womb or uterus. Okay, I am just kind of locating it first, and that is just my finger again. Okay, now you're going to feel the cold metal which I tried to warm up a little bit, but usually it's still cold. Is that okay?

Pt: Mm hmm.

Dr: Now I insert it just until I can see your cervix so that I can do the Pap test. Okay, now I can see your cervix very clearly now. . . .

Pt: Is that where I put the diaphragm?

Dr: Exactly, that is exactly where to put the diaphragm. Okay, now I am just using a soft brush to do the Pap test, okay?

Pt: Mm hmm.

Dr: And now I'm going to use one of those scrapes and sometimes you feel that scraping feeling, but usually what you feel is the pressure of the speculum being in place there. . . . Now I am just spraying those glass slides that I just took and that preserves them so they can be checked later. And now I am taking the speculum out. Are you still with me?

Pt: Yeah.

Dr: Now I am going to just check back inside your vagina, okay, and where my fingers are is where you put the diaphragm. Now I am going to ask you that when you go home you practice feeling where your cervix is. I am touching it right now. On you, it is a little bit off to your left side, okay, and it feels like the tip of your nose when you touch it. Okay. When I put one hand over here, between the two hands I can feel where your uterus is . . . And I am touching it right now and it feels normal. Now I am checking on each side for your ovaries. . . .

Pt: Can you feel all that?

Dr: Yes, I can feel all that, especially in someone like you, because you are very relaxed and I can feel everything. Okay, the next thing I am going to do is check your rectum and that will make you feel as though you have to have a bowel movement, right, that is just my finger in your rectum. That's kind of an uncomfortable feeling with some people. It feels completely normal.

Notice how the physician keeps talking, but frequently checks back with the patient, and is educating the patient all the while about her body and about the normality of the findings. Indeed, the proof that the technique is effective is in the patient's pleasure and wonderment ("Can you feel all that?") at the ability of a pelvic examination to tell a physician so much and at her ability to completely relax her muscles.

Your continued interview with the patient during the physical examination provides clarification and reassurance, and increases your efficiency. The new information aspect will gradually develop as you become more comfortable with the procedures of physical examination, so that concentration on the actual techniques can sink into the background and you are able to concentrate more thoroughly on your immediate observations. Until you are experienced, do not try to do the complete ROS during the physical examination. However, if you are looking at the eyes, for example, and this reminds you of an eye question you forgot to ask, go ahead and ask it. The physical examination is also a good time to chat with the patient, thereby finding out more about life and lifestyle. Such "small talk" yields pertinent information and also makes the patient more relaxed by distracting him or her from what your hands are doing.

Finally, the physical examination itself has not only a diagnostic but a therapeutic role. Simply touching the patient—the "laying on of hands"— may cause him or her to feel better and be reassured. Tactile communication opens up a channel of interpersonal response that can be very important in healing. In particular, specific attention to the painful areas of the body demonstrates that you have listened, understood, and are concerned about the patient's suffering.

ENDING THE INTERVIEW

When you have completed the physical examination, you reconvene the interview in order to terminate it. The goal of a good closure is no different from the goal of your entire interview and will be easier to attain if the patient understands from the outset the purpose of the interaction. The purpose will vary, depending on whether you are a student in a physical diagnosis course with a one-time shot at the patient, a clinical clerk following the patient for a short period, or a resident or attending physician with a long-term role in the patient's management. Overall, the patient should expect to feel understood and not be abused in any way. In history taking, this means that you have gotten the story straight and shown appropriate concern for his or her comfort, privacy, and modesty. The techniques of being accurate, empathic, respectful, and genuine apply to this part of the encounter as they do to all the other parts.

It is always a good idea to give the patient the opportunity to have the last word:

- "Anything else?"
- "Do you feel there is anything about what you have told me that I have not understood?"
- "Is there anything else you'd like to tell me or ask me?"

In your role as a student learning about medical interviewing or taking a physical diagnosis course, when you close any encounter with a patient you should:

- Provide a summary of what the patient has told you
- Be sure to let the patient have the last word or ask any additional questions
- Give a pleasant thank you and goodbye

This is fine with most patients, especially if you have been careful all along to clarify your role. If a patient asks a question you cannot answer about the disease or about his or her medical care, you should say something like "I am not able to answer that, but it is a good question to ask your doctor."

This is a truthful answer whether you are unable to answer because you do not know, or because, although you do know, the question is more properly answered by the patient's physician.

Once you have responsibility for a patient's care, the more typical closure implies a **contract** between you and the patient; it acknowledges responsibility for solving problems and providing care. In this general context, ending a patient encounter, whether it be a complete history and physical or a short office visit, should include these actions on the part of the clinician:

- **Differential diagnosis or hypotheses.** What you share depends on the patient—how sick he or she is, how knowledgeable, and whether or not he or she has other sources of information. What you share also depends on the illness; some findings are pertinent to the illness, while others are incidental or may be trivial. Avoid discussing what is interesting to you but may be irrelevant to the patient.

- **Devise a problem list with priorities.** This is painstaking and difficult at first but becomes easier with experience. It is important to realize that the physician's priorities often differ from those of the patient. Patients may be interested first in feeling better, second in their overall prognosis, and third in the specific diagnosis. Clinicians share these same concerns but often (especially while in medical school or in training) are more interested in making the diagnosis than in treating the symptoms. Treating the symptom is often not the same as treating the disease. Many trivial illnesses (e.g., simple upper respiratory tract infections) do not in themselves need specific medications but have symptoms that patients want treated. On the other hand, many significant illnesses (e.g., hypertension) have no symptoms but demand, from the doctor's point of view, specific therapy.

- **Agree on a plan of action and clarify responsibilities.** Determine what will happen next and who will do what. The physician may agree to order and interpret tests, talk with consultants, write prescriptions, or do procedures or an additional history and physical. The patient may agree to take the medication, modify diet, keep the follow-up appointment, or report further symptoms. Responsibilities are often blurred, especially in the patient who says, "I'm in your hands, Doc." Ideally, medical care is a partnership in which you negotiate an agreement or contract with the patient, but the character of that contract depends on the patient's illness (emergency care versus chronic antihypertensive therapy) and on the patient's acceptance of responsibility (see negotiation, Chap. 15).

- **Educate the patient.** The physician should tell the patient as much as the physician knows about the problem, within the limits of what the patient wants to know and can accept and understand. This is easier to say than to do and is a process over time as the physician learns about the patient and his or her problems. It is different for each physician, each patient, and each illness.

To conclude this chapter, here is an example of the closing minutes of an office visit (with a patient who suffers from back pain):

Dr: I don't find anything on my exam. I don't find anything that makes me think you have a pinched nerve. I think periodically you may be getting some nerve irritation and that's accounting for the pain that's shooting down your legs. What I think we should do, I want to check your x-rays that you had. I want to review those. I think we should prescribe bed rest for a while and just get you off of your feet. At least for a short time. Maybe 2, 3, or 4 days. Is that, are you able to do that?

Pt: Yeah.

Dr: You don't live by yourself?

Pt: No. I live with my daughter.

Dr: Okay, fine. I'm going to give you a couple of different medicines. I'll refill the Darvocets, but I only want you to use that as needed. I'm going to give you another medicine called Motrin. Are you able to take aspirin?

Pt: Yes.

Dr: So, I'm going to give you Motrin, which is an anti-inflammatory medicine. I don't want you to expect any overnight relief from the Motrin, because it takes several days, sometimes up to a week. So I'm going to give you the Motrin, Darvocet, and I'll give you a prescription for something called Pericolace, which is a very mild laxative and stool softener to make sure while you're . . . while you're down in bed rest that you don't get constipated. Do you have a heating pad at home?

Pt: Yeah, I have a moist heating pad.

Dr: Wonderful. You can use that every hour if you like, but I don't want you using it for more than 20 minutes at a time. But you can use it up to 20 minutes out of every hour. All right? So, I want you to really cut down on your activity—actually stay in bed for a couple of days, then gradually increase your activity. But no prolonged sitting or standing, and no bending or heavy lifting. I want to see you next week, preferably on Friday.

Pt: What about my physical therapy?

Dr: I want to lay off that for now.

Pt: Now will you explain to me again what the Motrin is?

Dr: Motrin is an anti-inflammatory drug. It's an arthritic drug.

Pt: In other words, it's supposed to help the pain in the back?

Dr: A lot of the pain in back injuries is due to irritation of the tissues and this will quiet down that irritation of the tissues, that in conjunction with, first of all, the rest. I didn't feel too much muscle spasm in your back now.

Pt: Well, that has quieted down some. I had quite a bit in October. It sort of quit, but I still have the pain.

Dr: There's your prescriptions, here's the Darvocets, only take that as needed for extra pain. The Motrin I want you to take one, four times per day: breakfast, lunch, dinner, bedtime, and you should take that continuously . . . I want to see you next week, preferably on Friday, that will give us a full week. Okay? And we will see in a week, see how you are doing and, as I said, in the meantime, I'll review the x-rays. Okay? Anything else?

Pt: I wanted to mention to you. I had gone for a Pap smear and they said the Pap smear was normal, I mean I don't have cancer. . . .

Notice how the physician shares the findings and clarifies the plan of action, including what the physician will do and expects the patient to do. Note, too, how the patient at the last minute brings up her concern about cancer possibly being the cause of her pain. The physician can now offer her appropriate reassurance that the etiology of her pain is not cancer; moreover, the physician will know that the patient's fear of cancer may reappear if the pain does not improve. It is not at all unusual for critical information like this to surface at the close of the interview when the patient feels comfortable and can see that he or she is being listened to. It is vital, therefore, that you demonstrate your open-ended attitude even as you close the encounter, as this physician did with the remark "Okay? Anything else?"

S U M M A R Y : The ROS, Physical Examination, and Closure

The objectives of the ROS are to:
- Identify active problems not yet discussed
- Associate additional symptoms with current illness

The ROS may occur late in the interview or, in part, during the physical examination, at which time you chat with the patient in order to:
- Obtain more ROS-type information
- Learn more about the patient as a person
- Make the patient more comfortable.

After the examination, you close the clinical encounter by:
- Summarizing what you heard and what you found
- Devising a problem list and negotiating priorities

- Outlining a plan of action and responsibilities
- Continuing to educate the patient

References

1. Platt FW, McMath JC. Clinical hypocompetence: The interview. *Ann Intern Med* 1979; 91:898–902.
2. Eisenberg L, Kleinman A. Clinical social science. In: Eisenberg L, Kleinman A, eds: *The Relevance of Social Science to Medicine*. Dordrecht, Holland, D. Reidel, 1980.

Suggested Readings

Novack DH. Therapeutic aspects of the clinical encounter. *J Gen Intern Med* 1987; 2:346–355.
Older J. Teaching touch at medical school. *JAMA* 1984; 252:931–933.

CHAPTER 7

I Shall Enumerate
Them to You

• • •

GETTING IT ALL DOWN AND
COMMUNICATING TO
OTHERS

At least I have a grip of the essential facts of the case. I shall
enumerate them to you, for nothing clears up a case so much
as stating it to another person.

Arthur Conan Doyle, Sherlock Holmes to Dr. Watson, "Silver Blaze"

After you have interviewed and examined your patient, you walk away,
perhaps carrying pages of cryptic and chaotic notes. You have the story
firmly, or perhaps not so firmly, in your head, as well as a few inklings of a
differential diagnosis. The most important part of your patient's work-up is
complete at this point, but before progressing further, you must put together
the story on paper, or "do the write-up." From the morass of your patient's
symptoms and experiences, what do you choose to include in the permanent
medical record? And how do you structure the story to make it most useful?

Because this text is limited to the skills of medical interviewing, in this
chapter we focus on how to conceptualize, format, and write down the medical history. However, the medical record is, in fact, a literary genre with its
own objectives and standards of practice. In this genre, a patient history
does not normally stand alone. Its proper format also includes physical and

laboratory data, an assessment or formulation (e.g., what the clinician's hypotheses are), and a plan for diagnosis and/or therapy, not to mention subsequent entries like flow sheets and progress notes. Consequently, to give a more complete picture of the medical record, we also present some guidelines for the other, nonhistory elements of your write-up.

This chapter consists of four major sections. In the first, we consider a few basic concepts about recording the written history. Whose story is it, the doctor's or the patient's? Then we consider the purposes of a medical record. The third section presents a basic outline for constructing the written history and physical examination. Finally, we consider the problem-oriented method of medical record keeping, commenting on some of its advantages and disadvantages.

WHAT GOES INTO THE WRITTEN HISTORY

Just the Facts?

Recording the history is not a question of "just the facts, ma'am." It is the end product of a long process of selection, interpretation, and editing. What you write on paper is a result of at least four levels of selection and interpretation.

- The first level is the patient's experience, or raw data—that is, the "facts" as they actually happened and what it was like to feel the throbbing headache or experience the room spinning around.
- The second level is the patient's conceptualization of the experience— that is, how the patient organizes the facts to construct a story that lends meaning and coherence to the experience. This conceptualization draws on the patient's values and beliefs. He or she began to weave this story even before seeking medical help, but your questions and selective attention helped create the current version.
- A third level is the clinical tale, the story you generate by means of the medical interview. Because you speak a medical language and live in a medical culture, you are able to reconstruct the patient's story so that it has some new "characters" (e.g., groupings of symptoms) and a somewhat different plot development.
- Finally, you select some of this story to record in the chart as the "write up." To do this, you apply certain canons of literary form. There are rules and guidelines appropriate to the write-up, just as there are rules and guidelines appropriate to other literary genres such as the short story or the nonfiction essay.

When we call the final product the medical history, it is easy to forget the interpretive and selective process that goes into producing it. The physician is not simply a passive secretary or scribe. It is both inefficient and virtually impossible to repeat everything the patient says. In this respect, it is useful to use the metaphor "interpreting a text" to describe diagnosis and problem solving in the physician-patient interaction.[1] This metaphor serves to highlight important features of medical practice that are obscured when we think of medicine as "hard" science (another metaphor!) and diagnosis as an exercise in logic or decision analysis.

What does all this mean? What seems at first glance to be "just the facts" is actually an interpretation of the facts. You are trying to understand the meaning of the patient's story, much as a literary critic tries to understand a text. The quality of your interpretation depends on your skill and experience, as well as the text's underlying readability. The context in which you see a patient or read a sentence can be a major determinant in your interpretation. No single interpretation of a book or of a patient's illness is final; there should be continuous re-evaluation. In medicine, as in literary criticism, a "true" interpretation is validated through open discourse among peers and consultants.

Recording Personal Information

Because we tend to believe that what is written in the chart is prima facie true, and because the medical record has so many functions, the record can become a powerful source of misinformation. Errors, such as mistakes in observation or clinical judgment, tend to be perpetuated because so much emphasis is placed on the written word. A wrong diagnosis or a judgmental remark, once written, is difficult to eradicate. Keep this issue in mind, particularly when recording personal data about the patient.

What personal data should be recorded? Here are some guidelines that attempt to steer between the Scylla of a biochemical approach to the patient and the Charybdis of disrespect or sentimentality.

- Be cautious about recording data about the patient's attitude, style, expectations, or health belief system. Although it is always useful to have relevant knowledge of this sort about the patient, it is not always important to write it explicitly. Unless a patient's dramatic or dependent style is out of the ordinary range, privacy and efficiency dictate silence. If you need to communicate a patient's style or idiosyncratic beliefs to others because they play a significant role in patient care, then the information should be written in a descriptive, as opposed to a judgmental, way.

- Delete certain personal information from the written record, such as explicit descriptions of sexual habits, problematic relationships, and criminal records, even if it may seem important. Imagining the chart being read by the patient is a useful criterion for what is appropriate to write.

- Include the patient's own words whenever possible, not just in the chief complaint. For example, recording that the patient describes the headache as "a deep pain like someone is twisting a screwdriver inside my brain" tells a lot about the patient and is less judgmental than writing "patient describes the headache in a bizarre fashion" or "patient is histrionic."

- Minimize distortion by avoiding language that "pathologizes." In medicine we often use words that turn people, experiences, or feelings into "pathologies."[3,4] The plain language of human experience does not seem medical enough for us. We like to use "depressed" rather than "sad," and rarely do we describe patients as "discouraged" or "courageous." To make the record more personally descriptive, avoid words like apathy, anxiety, denial, depression, and manipulative. Try instead to use words like determined, discouraged, hopeful, optimistic, brave, fearful, sad, or hopeless.

- Use behavioral or functional descriptions to convey personal information. By simply describing how the patient spends his or her day, what his or her hobbies are, or what he or she does on weekends, you can sketch important features of the person without getting too personal. Such statements fit well into the medical record; the operative principle is to be descriptive, not judgmental.

Another helpful way to look at the job of writing a medical history is to see yourself as an editor. The physician uses conventions and rules to create a case history out of the sprawling first draft presented by the patient. Form follows function. The rules ensure that the medical record will accomplish its goals efficiently and effectively. But what are these goals? What purposes does a permanent medical record serve?

FUNCTIONS OF THE MEDICAL RECORD

- **Memory aid.** Originally the medical record served only as a stimulus to jog a clinician's memory. Physicians kept brief notes on index cards. The complete information, though, was not on the card, but in the physician's mind. That is where clinical understanding and integration took place. Although today we have more extensive (and sometimes computerized) written records, we remember many details about our patients' lives and experiences that we do not write down, and we *think* many things that we dare not write down.

- **Communication.** The medical record, although mostly a memory aid, also serves to communicate with other health professionals. In the modern hospital or clinic setting, health care is a team activity; perhaps 50 or more people have legitimate access to an inpatient chart. Most of them will want to communicate their findings and their treatments to other members of the team. This communicative function leads to certain conventions regarding which observations are important to record and the form in which they ought to be recorded. The need to communicate also raises important questions about confidentiality. There is, after all, information about your patient that might be helpful to you as the primary physician, but which need not or should not be communicated to others, even if they are also members of the health-care team.

- **Quality assessment and research.** An attending physician evaluates his or her students and residents, at least in part, on the basis of their patient records. Hospital quality assurance and utilization review committees monitor the performance of physicians by reviewing their charts. The medical record also serves as a data source for clinical research. Retrospective chart reviews still serve as the backbone of clinical epidemiology, even though variations in available data, recording styles, and legibility present great methodologic problems.

- **Legal and administrative matters.** Insurance companies and managed-care programs use the chart to verify diagnosis and to establish that specific services were provided. Quality control and cost-containment strategies require that charts be reviewed and decisions be made partly on the basis of recorded data. Finally, the medical record is a written document that can be used as evidence in court.

FORMAT OF THE MEDICAL RECORD

Table 7–1 presents elements usually contained in a medical write-up. Although there is broad consensus on these major features, detailed conventions about the way they are put together vary from hospital to hospital,

TABLE 7–1   ELEMENTS OF MEDICAL CASE DESCRIPTION

Subjective
  History
    Identifying data
    Chief complaint: *Use the patient's own words.*
    History of the present illness: *Organize the story.*
    Other active problems: *Outline what else is going on.*
    Past medical history: *Note hospitalizations, surgery, allergies, important illnesses.*
    Family history: *Use a genogram or table.*
    Patient profile: *Sketch with care.*
    Review of systems: *Record significant positives and negatives.*

Objective
  Physical examination
  Laboratory data

Integrative
  Assessment: *The problem list*
  Plan

clinic to clinic, and practice to practice. Some institutions provide structured forms to use, at least for the more "objective" parts of the write-up, such as problem lists and physical examination; some have created paperless computerized records; and others still rely on old-fashioned lined paper. The following discussion is a relatively generic one into which most institution-specific formats should fit.

Identifying Data and Chief Complaint

The write-up begins with a succinct statement that identifies the patient and tells why he or she is seeking medical help. Often the patient's chief complaint, stated in the patient's own words, is the most effective descriptive statement to use. For example:

- Mr. Steven Maringo is a 47-year-old construction worker who came in because "I've had a sore throat for a month and it won't go away."
- Ms. Alice York is a 41-year-old chemist at Alcoa, with a history of "ulcers," who came in now because "I've had a burning pain under my ribs all week."
- Beth Salisbury is a 10-year-old fourth grader who came in because "my ear hurts" since yesterday.
- Mr. Fred Jones is a 32-year-old computer programmer referred by Dr. A. Zinger for evaluation of a persistent "washed-out feeling" and lower extremity weakness.

When a patient has been referred, as in the last example, it is important to record that fact. The patient may not have a chief complaint as such; he or she may be coming for a routine checkup or for a driver's license examination. Whatever the reason, it should be recorded in the patient's own words.

Other particularly relevant data also may be included in the introductory statement. For example, "Mr. Fred Jones is a 32-year-old, unmarried, African-American computer programmer who works at Ibex Industries. . . ." One should not try to pack this sentence with too many identifying features, however. Is the fact that Jones is unmarried or African-American relevant to his persistent "washed-out feeling"? Perhaps so. But a thousand other features might be relevant as well. It is best to strive for simplicity here, but many institutions have their own conventions about how to begin the write-up. Some, for example, might insist that all patients be identified by race and occupation, in addition to age and gender, no matter what their medical problems are.

Present Illness

This section should reflect your interpretation and organization of the patient's story. Although the diagnoses may be in doubt, you should have a good grasp of the patient's problem(s), and organize the **present illness** description accordingly. The description should be succinct, with emphasis on:

- Time course
- Symptom characteristics
- Functional deficits

Use the patient's own words and voice when possible, but remember that *you* are the author here. If the patient rambles or has 13 different complaints, that is no reason for you to ramble also or to produce an overly long present illness section. Your organization and choice of material should reflect your thinking about how the symptoms fit together, not the patient's.

For example, consider the transcription of an opening statement presented in Chapter 3 (p. 46). The written Present Illness section might begin thus:

> Mrs. P has been feeling "tired" and "worn out" even when she gets as much as 11 hours' sleep. Her sleep is interrupted by "hot flashes," although these are less frequent than they were previously.

The writer may choose to put the patient's concerns about nervousness and loss of libido under the Other Active Problems section (discussed later), or may include them in the Present Illness, if he or she considers them part of the same problem (a depressive disorder, for example).

You will frequently encounter patients who have had multiple hospital admissions and specialty consultations, and who have records an inch thick—perhaps someone with ischemic cardiomyopathy and obstructive pulmonary disease who frequently requires emergency care, or a patient with metastatic breast cancer, admitted numerous times for courses of chemotherapy. It is tempting to construct the "present history" of such a patient from old chart data, with little input from the patient himself or herself. For example:

> Mrs. Ely was first found to have carcinoma of the breast in May 1990, after which she underwent a left simple mastectomy, followed by a course of local irradiation. In June 1993 she was noted to have bone metastases in T4 and L1 . . . (a series of medical interventions) . . . and today (in November 1996) is admitted to be evaluated for further chemotherapy.

This is not a history of an illness; it is a chronicle of medical events. Does the patient currently have symptoms? Why is chemotherapy being considered at this point in time, rather than last year or next month? The patient's voice is absent. Medical records can provide supplemental information that sheds light on the current problem, but it is never appropriate to construct a narrative based only on data from old records and call it "present illness."

Other Active Medical Problems

It is useful to consider this a separate section, although sometimes it may be integrated with the Present Illness section. Patients often have complex and chronic medical problems. A given episode of illness may well be an exacerbation of a chronic problem, or interact with another ongoing disease. Because of this, it is important to select continuing problems from the Past Medical History and to provide details about their current status. In the previous example, if Mrs. Ely had been admitted for symptoms of pneumonia, her history of breast cancer and chemotherapy would certainly be relevant, and it should be recorded thoroughly in this part of the text.

Past Medical History

This section begins the more standardized or routine part of the write-up. By definition, it includes only those problems not directly (or obviously) relevant to the illness at hand. The format, as described in Chapter 4, should be as follows:

- Serious illnesses, from childhood to the present, including hospitalizations
- Surgical procedures
- Accidents and injuries
- Pregnancies, deliveries, and complications
- Allergies, including type and known allergens
- Current medications, including over-the-counter drugs, with dosages and schedule (these may also be listed under Other Active Problems)
- Health maintenance data, including immunizations and screening tests

Family History

The **family history** is best presented in a genogram that shows relationships in a diagrammatic form (Fig. 7–1). Squares represent males, circles females. A diagonal line or "x" indicates that the person has died. Diseases may be indicated above or below the symbols. Alternatively, the family history can be presented in tabular form. This method is more efficient if the patient does not have much medical information about his or her family. Relationships can be indicated by abbreviations; for example, MGM for maternal grandmother, PGF for paternal grandfather, and so forth. Such a family history might look like:

- MGM (d. age 60s), unknown cause
- MGF (d. age 70), heart attack
- PGF (92), arthritis, forgetful

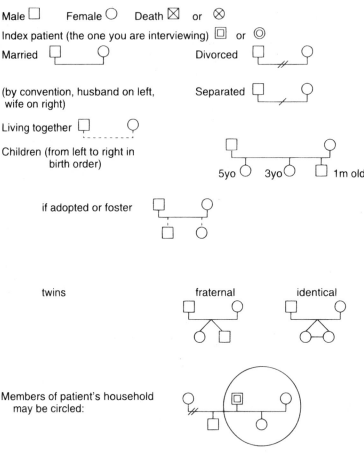

FIGURE 7–1 Family history: the genogram.

Social History and Patient Profile

The object of the **patient profile** is to give a picture of the patient as a functioning person and to record medically related or health-related behavior. The harried physician should avoid making the person invisible and recording only whether he or she smokes tobacco or drinks alcohol. On the other hand, the writer should also avoid becoming too discursive or personal. Approach writing the Patient Profile with a standard outline in mind, similar to the outline used during your interview, even though, in a given case, you need not necessarily write something for each item:

- Brief biography (e.g., place of birth, education, military service, and years in this locality)
- Current marital, family, and home situation

- Occupation and occupational history, including toxic exposures and stresses
- Lifestyle (e.g., religious affiliation, personal interests, hobbies, travel, and exercise)
- Diet and nutrition
- Personal habits (e.g., use of tobacco, alcohol, and "recreational" drugs)
- A typical day's activities (this may be placed under Present Illness when a change in functional status is an important descriptor of the illness)
- Relevant feelings and beliefs (e.g., work satisfaction, perceived stresses, understanding of the illness, and attitudes toward health care)

Review of Systems

Data obtained in the **review of systems** (ROS) section of the interview may be incorporated into the written Present Illness, if relevant to the current problem; placed in a structured system-by-system ROS section; or simply left unwritten.

Beginners should include a fairly comprehensive ROS to develop the discipline of considering each system in turn. More experienced clinicians will usually write a few positive findings and pertinent negative findings. They will then indicate that the rest of the ROS was "unremarkable" or "negative."

Physical Examination

Although there are many local variations, the overall format is standard. You begin with a statement about the patient's general appearance and continue with vital signs (respiratory rate, blood pressure, pulse rate, and temperature) and the results of the examination of skin, head, eyes, ears, nose, throat, neck, lymphatic system, chest, back, breasts, heart, abdomen, rectum, genitourinary system, extremities, musculoskeletal system, nervous system, and, finally, mental status. Though mental status data are generally collected by talking as opposed to touching, they are recorded as part of the physical examination.

Laboratory Work

Results of diagnostic studies may be included as part of the initial write-up if they are routine, or are available shortly after your interview and physical examination. In such cases, the results are part of the database upon which your assessment and plan are based. There is no standard method of recording laboratory or x-ray findings. Perhaps the most efficient and efficacious way is to use appropriate flow sheets and not place these data in the midst of written text. Nevertheless, it can be useful to have a snapshot of basic studies (complete blood count and differential, urinalysis, serum chemistries, chest x-ray, or electrocardiogram) in the database to help buttress your initial assessment. Each institution has its own recommended set of routine laboratory work for new patients, or for patients admitted to the hospital. In recent years, however, the emphasis has been on selecting diagnostic studies, rather than on ordering "routine" studies.

Assessment and Plan

The best way of organizing your assessment and plan is to use principles derived from the problem-oriented medical record system, which we will now address in some detail.

PROBLEM-ORIENTED RECORDS

In 1970, Lawrence Weed[2] introduced the **problem-oriented medical record** (POMR), and this approach has had widespread acceptance during the ensuing decades. The main elements of the POMR system are:

- A database that includes the written history, physical examination, and laboratory data
- A problem list that displays the names of all identified problems, not simply medical diagnoses; this list includes both current and inactive problems, and is updated regularly
- A standard format for writing about each problem in one's own formulation or in daily progress notes, which requires that a note be divided into four sections (hence, the acronym **SOAP notes** or **SOAP format**)
  - Subjective, recounting symptoms and personal data
  - Objective, dealing with physical signs and laboratory data
  - Assessment, expressing the clinician's analysis of the problem
  - Plan, stating the measures to be taken
- Devices such as flow sheets to simplify, organize, and display data

One main thrust of the problem-oriented system was to humanize medical care by focusing attention on the patient's perceived problems, rather than solely on standard medical diagnoses. For example, symptoms like "abdominal pain" or "swollen elbow" are perfectly appropriate to list as problems in an initial evaluation. Subsequently, the patient might be found to suffer from irritable bowel syndrome, which would then explain the abdominal pain and replace the words "abdominal pain" on the problem list. Alternatively, the patient might be found to have inflammatory bowel disease with an associated arthritis. This diagnosis could explain two problems, abdominal discomfort and swelling of the elbow. Frequently, however, the clinician might find no ready diagnostic explanation; then, even though no diagnosis is made, the symptom is still a "problem."

In Weed's formulation, problems also could be personal, social, financial, or functional difficulties, not just somatic symptoms or medical disorders. Poor vision, unemployment, marital discord, and cigarette smoking are all separate problems, some of which are amenable to the traditional method of differential diagnosis and some of which are not. Because a separate SOAP note was supposed to be written for each problem, the Weed system forced the physician to address each problem on a regular basis and not let some of them fall between the cracks. Including separate sections for subjective and objective data was also intended to humanize clinical practice by forcing physicians to take subjective data seriously. The patient's feelings and concerns had to be considered, written in the note, and presumably used in making the assessment.

The difficulties with POMR are both structural and cultural. The structural concern is that the system is cumbersome. Today, only the sickest and most complicated patients are hospitalized, and they often have six or eight active problems. It is difficult and time- and space-consuming to write a daily SOAP note on each one. In the office setting, patients may also have numerous problems, and the clinician has even less time for charting.

The cultural difficulty is that, given our disease-oriented medical culture, we tend to restrict the patient's problems to medical diagnoses, thus losing the system's main advantage. Students and interns may write elaborate SOAP notes on diabetes, but they rarely indicate that marital discord is an active problem and they almost certainly never SOAP it. Moreover, the subjective category, rather than emphasizing the critical importance of patient stories, as it was intended to do, plays second fiddle to the objective category. We treat subjective data as less scientific—and, therefore, less worthy—than objective data. Often problems are discussed in SOAP notes with no entry under "subjective" at all.

We subscribe to the Weed philosophy and believe that (at a minimum) the clinician should incorporate the following features in medical write-ups and records:

- Develop a well-rounded database on each patient. The database should include a patient narrative that reflects the patient's personality. It may be written over a period of time, however, and need not (should not) be a one-shot database.

- Think in broad human terms when identifying problems and include the types of situations and disabilities that Weed originally intended. This means that a symptom or a situation that constitutes a problem for the patient should be listed, even if you cannot comfortably fit it into a diagnosis.

- Keep a complete, frequently revised problem list on each patient.
- Respect subjective data and use them regularly in writing progress notes. The term "person-oriented" is perhaps more appropriate than "subjective"; remember that many of our "objective" data are heavily encrusted with interpretation and, therefore, are also in a sense subjective.
- Use flow sheets and other devices to jog your memory, organize complex data, and enhance patient care.

S U M M A R Y : The Clinical Narrative

In this chapter we presented various considerations involved in translating your interview experience (and notes) into a written case "write-up." The "write-up" and other parts of the medical record serve as memory aids, methods of communication, data for quality assessment and research, and legal or administrative documents. A typical format for the case description is outlined in Table 7–1.

We also discussed a number of additional points about clinical narratives and medical records:

- The Present Illness section is a narrative of the patient's experience; it should read like a story.

- When recording personal information, be careful to respect the patient's privacy as much as possible, and use language that describes but does not pathologize.

- The problem-based medical record system includes several useful concepts that enhance patient care:
  - The initial database
  - A broad human perspective, rather than a narrow disease perspective
  - Problem lists
  - Respect for subjective data
  - Flow sheets

References

1. Gogel EL, Terry JS. Medicine as interpretation: The uses of literary metaphors and methods. *J Med Philos* 1987; 12:205–217.
2. Weed LL. *Medical Records, Medical Education, and Patient Care.* Cleveland, Case Western Reserve University Press, 1970.

3. Donnelly WJ. Righting the medical record. Transforming chronicle into story. *JAMA* 1988; 260:823–825.

4. Donnelly WJ. Medical language as symptom: Doctor talk in teaching hospitals. *Perspect Biol Med* 1986; 30:81–94.

Suggested Reading

Hawkins AH. *Reconstructing Illness. Studies in Pathography.* West Lafayette, IN, Purdue University Press, 1993.

Hunter KM. *Doctors' Stories. The Narrative Structure of Medical Knowledge.* Princeton, NJ, Princeton University Press, 1991.

PART TWO

BASIC SKILLS IN PRACTICE: APPLYING THE PATIENT'S STORY

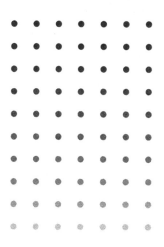

CHAPTER 8

A Different Silhouette

• • •

PEDIATRIC AND GERIATRIC INTERVIEWING

A human being sheds its leaves like a tree. Sickness prunes it down; and it no longer offers the same silhouette to the eyes which loved it, to the people to whom it afforded shade and comfort.

Edmond and Jules deGoncourt, Journal, July 22, 1862

In the first seven chapters, we presented basic skills of medical interviewing and what might be called a "generic" version of the medical history. In clinical practice, you often have to adapt the interview to meet the needs of particular groups of patients or specific patient-care situations. The brief and highly focused history given by a trauma patient in the emergency department is very different in both style and content from the multifaceted history obtained from a patient being evaluated for chronic illness. In this chapter, we consider how to adapt your interview to patients in the extremes of the age spectrum—namely, children and older persons.

THE PEDIATRIC PATIENT*

Why devote a separate section to pediatric interviewing? Are the medical histories of children so different from those of adults? In the following pages, we take the perspective that children and adolescents are not merely "miniature adults." Not only is the style of a pediatric interview different from the medical history elicited from an adult, but the style of the pediatric interview also varies dynamically from one developmental stage of childhood to the next.

Children versus Grown-ups: Similarities and Differences

There are, of course, many similarities between pediatric and adult medical interviews. For example, the basic organization of a clinical history is the same for patients of all ages: chief complaint, history of present illness, past medical history, family history, patient profile, and review of systems. Similarly, skills and values that facilitate good adult patient-clinician interactions, such as empathy, respect, and confidentiality, are equally important in pediatrics.

The two most important differences between the adult and pediatric interview are the individuals who participate in the conversation and the topics that are emphasized at a particular stage of development. With regard to the participants, for example, parents or other family members, instead of or in addition to the patient, must often provide information. Although this need is obvious in the case of a preverbal child, potential problems arise in gathering information, and the precise point at which a verbal child has the skill to contribute his or her own history is not always easy to determine. With regard to topics, the prenatal history, for example, is vitally important in the case of a neonate but less so in the case of an adolescent. And the achievement of developmental milestones, while critical to the routine assessment of a 6-month-old, is of minimal significance in the evaluation of a "straight As" second grader who presents with a sore throat.

Setting the Stage for Effective Communication

Even the most precise, empathic historian needs a private and comfortable environment. If the patient is in a hospital room that contains several beds, the neighbor's television is playing, visitors are chatting, and medical personnel are performing procedures, then families will feel uncomfortable even talking about mundane historical items, much less giving thoughtful observations of behavior or potentially embarrassing details. Before starting, you should insist that the television and radio be turned off. If possible, room-

---

*The pediatric section in Edition 2 was co-authored by Kenneth Schuitt, MD.

mates may be taken elsewhere by their parents or by staff members. Otherwise, curtains should be drawn around the child's bed to provide at least the illusion of privacy. Similarly, you should see that a neonate is comfortable and quiet before expecting his or her parents to be relaxed enough to provide you with detailed information. In the case of a preschool child, offering the patient a toy to occupy his or her attention may well improve the efficiency of an interview. Spend a few moments at the beginning of an interview with a newborn's parents to admire the baby, with a 2-year-old's mother to charm the toddler, or with a school child to query him or her about a favorite television show or hobby. With children it is often easier to establish rapport indirectly by admiring a toy or a pair of new shoes as opposed to an (overly) enthusiastic greeting to the child himself. Then, spend a few moments talking to the parent or guardian to give the child time to size you up (while you size up the child out of the corner of your eye).

You should make no assumptions and certainly no judgments about the relationship of the caretaking adults to the child patient. The parents of an infant may not necessarily bear the same married name. Thus, the term "his father" rather than "your husband" or "the baby's mother" rather than "your wife" might be more appropriate until the parental relationship is better understood. Similarly, an infant and his or her parent may not carry the same surname. A brief glance at the registration form might reveal that the infant's name is Doe, while the mother's and father's name is Smith. Because you need to understand the relationship for the benefit of the child, it is best to ask, simply and nonjudgmentally, "I notice that your name is Smith and William's name is Doe. Can you explain the relationship to me?"

Finally, try to tailor your vocabulary to the level of understanding of the family members with whom you are speaking. Discernment of their sophistication is subject to bias and may at times be difficult. One senior pediatric faculty member, who frequently berated his students for ignoring education and background when talking to parents, was asked to see a child whose mother and father were plainly dressed and who came from a rural part of the state. Following his own admonition, he began speaking very slowly and trying to use a quite simple vocabulary, only to discover that the father himself was a physician and the mother a nurse!

Talking with Patients of Different Ages

The style and content of a medical interview, as well as its participants, vary enormously with the child's age. The questions you ask new parents will be very different from those you ask a teenager. The content of the medical history changes with age just as the style and dynamics change. Topics that are obviously important in the prenatal visit or in the newborn interview become distinctly less important as the child matures and, indeed, may not be mentioned at all in the medical conversation with an adolescent. For convenience, we distinguish four types of pediatric medical history: the prenatal visit, the visit with the infant or toddler, the visit with the school-age child, and, finally, the visit with the adolescent.

THE PRENATAL VISIT

Ideally, the person who will be responsible for the medical care of a newborn should meet with the prospective parents. The **prenatal visit** allows the caregiver to obtain important medical information, and establishes a partnership of mutual trust and respect. The diminished role of extended, multigenerational families means that in many cases the emotional and educational support for new parents may come from a physician or nurse, rather than from their parents and siblings. A brief informal meeting can initiate such a support system and dispel myths and preconceptions that the potential parents might have. The information you acquire during this prenatal visit includes a detailed family history; plans for feeding the baby (breast versus bottle); circumcision (yes or no); and the parents' knowledge about child care. Practical issues like the schedule for well-child office visits, medical fees, and telephone access also can be presented at this time.

During your meeting with prospective parents, obtain information about the family history: familial disease, previous histories of birth defects, and perinatal deaths. The purpose of this family history is twofold:

- To alert you to possible genetic disease in the infant
- To reassure or inform parents concerned about implications for their child of certain familial illnesses or tendencies

Listen especially for details of miscarriages and neonatal or childhood illness or death. The parents' health and their past medical history should be outlined in some detail, especially with respect to disease states that might endanger the life or health of the fetus during pregnancy. Pay attention to the physical, social, and emotional environment into which the child will be born. Parents' discussion of their plans for feeding the baby and their knowledge of child care will direct your educational efforts.

This prenatal interaction also provides an opportunity to give some anticipatory guidance to parents. For example, take the opportunity to discuss issues such as:

- The changes that will occur in parents' and siblings' lives with the newborn's arrival
- Identification of support persons for the mother and father when the infant goes home
- Information about safety for the infant at home and in the automobile
- Preparation of siblings for the new addition to their family

THE INFANT AND TODDLER

During infancy and the preschool years, the patient is the reason for the visit and the focus of the interview but not usually a participant in the interview. Although the patient may add little to the actual conversation, pediatric medicine is certainly not "akin to veterinary medicine," as some cynics would suggest! In most situations, you will conduct the interview while the infant or toddler is present, for several reasons. First, this small but important person serves as a catalyst to aid parents' recall of historical details. Second, parents are likely to be more comfortable if they are with their sick child, and certainly children will be more comfortable with their parents. Finally, in the case of preschool children, when the child sees you interacting with the mother or father, the child is more likely (very tentatively) to develop a feeling of trust.

If the infant is fussy or in pain, he or she will only distract both you and the parents. The situation might require a pacifier or bottle for the neonate or a familiar toy for the toddler. It is useful to carry around a colorful item or two to interest your preschool patients. Sometimes inexperienced clinicians will either ignore the patient completely (to the consternation of parents) or try to become instant "buddies" with the child, forgetting that usually by 1 year of age a child has become quite wary or even frightened of strangers. Moreover, illness may make the toddler irritable, and the clinical setting may be terrifying. A good compromise is to begin the encounter with a simple friendly greeting, followed by the enthusiastic but brief examination of one of the child's own toys rather than of the child himself or herself.

The medical history here must include information about the perinatal period:

- Complications and problems during the pregnancy
- Duration and complications of labor
- Problems during the infant's first days of life

If a family history has not already been obtained, you should take a careful family history as well. Crying, sleeping, and bowel and bladder function should be discussed. A careful review of developmental stages must be obtained, focusing on different milestones depending on the age of the child. Ascertain the child's immunization status, including reactions to the immunizations. Nutrition questions are also important in your clinical history. A few screening questions often suffice:

- "How many ounces of formula (or, for older children, milk) does your baby take each day?" For breast-fed babies, "How many times does the baby nurse in 24 hours?" and "What's the longest he or she goes between feedings?"

- For older infants and toddlers, "Are there any foods your child refuses to eat?"
- "Does your child get much in the way of sweets and junk food?"

Because anticipatory guidance plays an important role in every patient-family-doctor interaction in this age group, the clinician should obtain enough information that he or she can later discuss accident prevention, feeding, toilet training, and such developmental issues as teething and acquisition of normal speech patterns. The content of the interview varies with the reason for the visit: well-child care, an office visit for illness, or a very sick child or a child about to have a surgical procedure. The child's demeanor and the parents' level of anxiety and ability to provide precise information about the child's illness will vary. Parents may be very focused on whether they have cared for their child correctly or have done anything to provoke or worsen an illness. They will benefit from reassurance that they are good parents and have acted properly. Sometimes, especially early in the interview, you may be unable to provide such reassurance and may need to say:

> I understand your concern about whether you should have given Molly that cold medicine, but I'd like to leave that aside for the moment and get back to how she's been acting over the last few days. When did you first notice that she wasn't her usual self?

Once you have established the history, you will be able to reassure the parents that they have not hurt their child or, alternatively, to educate them in the proper care of a sick child.

The symptoms of pediatric illness, particularly in the preverbal child, are often nonspecific and tell us more about how sick the child is than precisely what the illness is. A 15-month-old cannot tell us that his or her left ear hurts; rather, he or she will cry, be irritable, have a fever, and possibly have a loss of appetite or even vomiting and diarrhea. If we are lucky, the child may tug at his left ear, but many children with healthy ears do that as well. We have to rely on our physical examination to make the diagnosis of left otitis media. But if the child is exceedingly irritable, refuses to play, and refuses liquids, we may need to rule out meningitis as well with additional diagnostic studies. Table 8–1 lists the key information required in the infant and toddler interview.

THE SCHOOL-AGE CHILD

When a child reaches the age of 5 or 6 years, the interactive balance in the interview begins to change. Children are then more able to contribute substantially to the collection of data, but their reports are usually broad and sometimes difficult to interpret. Thus, you must turn to parents to provide accuracy and precision, while always trying to confirm the data insofar as is possible with the small patient. An enormous maturational range is found

TABLE 8–1 CONTENT OF INFANT AND TODDLER INTERVIEW

Reason for Visit	Topics Discussed
Well-child visit	Parental concerns
	Dates of prior immunizations. Is child current?
	Prenatal and birth history
	Developmental milestones achieved
	Eruption of teeth
	Habits: sleeping, crying, and bowel and bladder function
	Intercurrent illness and other illnesses
	Nutrition history
	Cultural and family practices (feeding, taping umbilical hernias, keeping face covered to prevent colic, and so on)
Sick visit or admission to hospital	All of the topics discussed in a well-child visit
	History of Present Illness (Chap. 3) with special emphasis on time of onset, initial symptoms, and subsequent symptoms
	Difficulty feeding—too slow, not at all, refusal of liquids, refusal of solids, or preference for water or juice as opposed to milk or formula
	State of hydration
	Does the infant or child seem himself or herself?
	As playful, alert, and pleasant as usual? Acting sick?
	Temperature taken at home? rectal? axillary?
	Medications (including over-the-counter medications) already given and their dosages?
	What concerns the parents most? What do they think is causing illness?
	History of recent similar illnesses in patient or family?

in elementary school-age children. You can expect to find behaviors ranging from shy, sullen, and silent to that of the garrulous child who cannot be stopped! Thus, as a sensitive historian, you must take your cues from observing the patient before deciding whether and how much to involve the child in actual history taking.

In general, the school-age child is a healthy child. In addition to obtaining historical information concerning immunizations, development, and nutrition, the psychosocial aspects of a child's history become more important during these years. Knowledge of the child's school performance and

TABLE 8–2   CONTENT OF SCHOOL-AGED CHILD INTERVIEW

Reason for Visit	Topics Discussed
Well-child visit	Parental concerns
	School progress, school readiness, relationships with peers
	Developmental milestones achieved? At what age?
	Habits (eating, sleeping, and continence)
	Age-appropriate play?
	Similarities to and differences from peers
	Significant past and birth history
	Illnesses since last visit
	Dates of prior immunizations
	Nutrition
Sick visit or admission to hospital	All of the topics discussed in well-child visit
	History of Present Illness (Chap. 3) with special emphasis on parent's observations
	Child's descriptions of symptoms
	Medications (including over-the-counter medication) already tried
	Similar illnesses in household or peer group

friends is necessary for the global understanding of a school-aged child's well-being. Anticipatory guidance at this age emphasizes accident prevention, both in the home and at school, and good nutrition. Special aspects of the content of the interview of the school-age child are indicated in Table 8–2.

THE ADOLESCENT

Your interactions with teenagers are potentially the most complicated and difficult of any interviews you will conduct. The adolescent person is frequently ambivalent or confused by his or her own feelings and resists talking about them. Moreover, during the adolescent years, patients take an increasingly active role in their own health care, while their parents move progressively into the background. This is a change that many mothers and fathers, as well as their teenage children, find difficult. You may initiate the interview with an unfamiliar teenager with a direct, unaffected introduction:

Dr: Hi, I'm Dr. Smith and I'm glad to meet you. Tell me what made you decide to come to see me or (as is often the case) what made your parents bring you?

Remember that initially you are a stranger and must establish a basis for trust. Many physicians try to become instant friends with teenagers, succeeding only in confusing or antagonizing them. It is appropriate to talk with adolescents alone for part of the interview, if not for the whole interaction. Most parents are cooperative and will leave the room without difficulty when you explain:

Dr: You know how important it is for you to feel that you have a private and confidential relationship with your doctor, and most of my young patients feel the same way. So I'm going to ask you to leave while I talk with Jamie. Is there anything you'd like to tell me before you go?

When speaking with an adolescent, establish that your conversation is confidential. Whether the information is potentially embarrassing or not, build trust by assuring the patient:

Dr: I always want to make it clear to all my patients that what they tell me is private. I will not repeat anything you say unless you give me permission to do so. But you know, your Mom cares about you and may have some concerns about what we do today. If she asks me anything, in order to protect your privacy, I'm going to tell her that she has to ask you. So you might want to think about what you'd like to tell her, and we can talk about that some more at the end of our visit.

This kind of statement not only respects the adolescent's desire for autonomy but also acknowledges the parents' rightful interest in their child who has not yet achieved full adult status. It also implies that parents and their children should talk about important things, even those that are difficult, such as sexuality.

The sexual history is a particularly difficult topic for adolescents. As with patients in any other age group, you should use clear language that the patient understands and proceed from less intimate questions ("Tell me about your family and friends." "Do you have any special friends?" "How about boyfriends or girlfriends?") to more intimate ones ("Do your friends go on dates?" "How do they feel about having sex?" "How do you feel?" "Are you sexually active now?").

One problem, of course, is making sure that when you use a term such as "sexually active," you are sure the patient understands what you mean. Young teenagers vary widely in their sexual knowledge and experience; among 14-year-old girls, you will find those who have already been pregnant and others who will look wide-eyed and disbelieving that you could even think of asking such questions. For this reason, questions about their peer group as well as questions that do not imply any right answer or particular level of experience are useful. For example:

Dr: Some girls your age who are late with their period will worry that they may have gotten pregnant. Have you had any worries like that?

Pt: No, because I know I can't be.

Dr: You can't be. Tell me more.

Pt: Well, I didn't have sex. I don't even go with boys; none of my friends do.

Sometimes the conversation takes a different turn:

Dr: Some girls your age who are late with their period will worry that they may have gotten pregnant. Have you had any worries like that?

Pt: Well, I thought about it.

Dr: Tell me more.

Pt: Well, I don't really think I can be.

Dr: Did he touch you or did he put his penis near you or inside you?

Notice the need to be simple and precise in your language so you can be sure that you are obtaining accurate information.

Important information to obtain from the teenager centers around the teenager's interaction with his or her environment and social world. Tactfully posed questions dealing with drugs and alcohol, sexuality, contraception, and sexually transmitted diseases are an important part of a medical history in this age group. But even the most tactful interviewer often has difficulty breaking through the outward reserve that many adolescents show. If this is the case, posing sensitive questions in the past tense is sometimes helpful. For example, rather than asking, "Do you smoke cigarettes?" you might ask, "Were you smoking cigarettes 6 months ago?" This avoids direct confrontation. Here is another example of how you might "open up" a silent and possibly angry adolescent interview:

Dr: I'm sorry that your father dragged you in here against your will. I know if I were in your shoes I'd be pretty angry. But since we have this time together, do you think we could talk about some of the things that have been going on in your life? None of this is any of my business unless it's okay with you for me to get to know you better. I'd like to hear more about how you've been feeling.

Other important issues to discover during the interview are:

- School performance
- The presence or absence of close friends
- Behavioral difficulties both at home and at school

Ideally, most of this information will be obtained directly from the adolescent rather than from a parent or guardian. Topics important to review during the visit with the adolescent patient are listed in Table 8–3.

THE ELDERLY PATIENT

In this part of the chapter, we consider some of the special sensitivities and skills required for effective interviewing of older or geriatric patients. Who are these "older" patients? Here is the opening exchange of a woman seeing

TABLE 8–3   CONTENT OF THE ADOLESCENT INTERVIEW

Reason for Visit	Topics Discussed
Well-child visit	Parental concerns and confidentiality in the doctor-patient relationship
	School progress and peer relationships
	Habits (eating, sleeping, physical activity)
	Smoking, alcohol and drug use
	Sexuality and sexual activity
	Past history (illnesses, medications, allergies)
	Interval history (any illness or symptoms since last visit)
	Immunizations (and related childhood diseases)
	Anticipatory guidance:
	Diet and exercise
	Injury prevention (bicycle, motor vehicle, firearms)
	Smoking, alcohol and drug use
	Sexuality, contraception, unintended pregnancies, STDs
	Stress, depression, hopelessness
Sick visit	Reason for coming (parent's view, adolescent's view)
	History of present illness and related review of systems
	Boundaries of confidentiality (what parent needs to know when adolescent is sick)
	Possible relationship of sexual activity and substance use to current symptoms
	An abbreviated review of well-visit topics if the sick visit is also a first visit to the office

STDs = sexually transmitted diseases.

her physician in the office for follow-up of hypertension and chronic diarrhea:

Dr: So how are you?
Pt: Okay, I guess. I guess it's just old age.
Dr: What about old age?

When does old age begin? This patient was 88 years old; but what if she had been only 78, 68, or 58? Although you should have special concerns if a 58-year-old woman or man complains of "old age," you will find it difficult to have any hard and fast rules about when an "older person" has become "old." The 68-year-old chief executive with neither health problems nor plans to retire is certainly not the same kind of older person as the 68-year-old retired mill worker with oxygen-dependent chronic lung disease and recent memory loss. The former would find questions about his ability to perform routine activities of daily living insulting if not bizarre; the latter would find such questions very relevant to his overall management. So the approach to older persons must be individualized and geared to the patient's stage of life, as opposed to making rigid classifications based on chronologic age.

Special aspects of history taking in this group include the style and content of the interview, mental status testing, and the problem of the "third party" in caring for elderly patients.

Style

The short vignette just presented illustrates the way in which many elderly patients attribute their symptoms to normal aging and may require open-ended prompting ("What do you mean by 'old age'?") to discuss symptoms that could indicate a specific disease process as opposed to senescence. Patients, for example, may attribute nocturia or joint pains to aging, even though these symptoms may, in fact, indicate specific diseases, such as heart failure or tendinitis. Moreover, vague symptoms may have special implications in the elderly, as in the case of a 90-year-old man with pneumonia who experiences loss of appetite and feelings of malaise rather than a more typical presentation with fever and cough. Likewise, chronic symptoms must be distinguished from acute or unstable symptoms. For example, the sudden onset of urinary incontinence requires a different approach than a report of incontinence of many years' duration. You also will notice that the pace of the interview is often slower and that the elderly infuse their medical stories with a lifetime of experience that demands and informs our respect. These are just some of the stylistic changes that you will note as you interview the geriatric patient.

Content

In addition to changes in style, the geriatric history emphasizes somewhat different content areas as well. For example, remote events, such as childhood history, are usually not relevant and may be obtained with a minimum amount of detail, like "Any unusual illnesses when you were a child?" The family history may assume less importance as well, because most familial diseases will have expressed themselves by the time a person reaches old age. The family history also takes on a different twist because you are now not only looking at the preceding generation but querying the elderly about their children and grandchildren as well. For example, an older woman whose daughter has breast cancer may herself be at increased risk of the disease and may not know that, in fact, it was breast cancer that took the life of her mother 40 years earlier. Moreover, elderly persons may worry about the health of their children and grandchildren, and your interest in their families provides an opportunity to explore those concerns.

Perhaps the most striking difference in the history of elderly patients is the need to assess their functional status in terms of everyday activities and their abilities to do those things necessary to sustain and enjoy life. The social history (or patient profile; see Chap. 5) includes most basic activities of daily living. Among these are the older person's ability to eat (chew and swallow), sleep, bathe, dress, walk or move about unaided, and maintain continence. Ability to cook and perform simple household chores also must be assessed. Several useful rating scales are available for measuring functional status or activities of daily living.[1]

Try to determine if the person is able to maintain a normal sleep-wake cycle; one useful question is "Are you able to sleep when you want to sleep and not sleep when you don't want to?" If bowel or bladder incontinence is a problem, you will need to get additional details such as the location of the bathroom and the patient's ease in getting there. Details about diet include the ability to afford, shop for, and prepare food, as well as some consideration of specific nutrients such as calcium (needed to prevent osteoporosis) and fiber (which may help prevent constipation and treat diverticular disease or hemorrhoids).

You should also assess sexual feelings and function, but this must be done sensitively and in context. Frail, sick, or widowed elderly patients may find questions like "Are you sexually active?" or "Are you having any sexual problems?" surprising, if not downright inappropriate. It is better to give the patient plenty of room to answer, based on his or her own situation. For example, "As people get older they sometimes find that their marriage changes. How has it been for you?" and then "Has anything changed in your sexual relationship?" Change in sexual function also may be related to specific illness, rather than to age per se. For example, "I can see that you're having problems with the circulation in your legs. Sometimes when men have this problem they also notice problems getting an erection. Have you noticed anything like that?"

Another content area of special importance in elderly persons is the detailed review of all medications—over-the-counter as well as prescription drugs. This is best accomplished by asking patients to bring all their pill containers with them, even the containers of drugs they no longer take. Finally, immunization status, including diphtheria-tetanus, influenza, and pneumococcal vaccines, and any adverse reactions to these immunizations, is an important part of the geriatric history that often is given insufficient attention.

Mental Status Assessment

The interviewer must facilitate a technically competent interview with patients who may be frail, hard of hearing, visually impaired, or suffering from memory loss. You should quickly and inconspicuously assess cognitive function in the opening moments of the interview, usually without a formal mental status examination. The purpose of this informal assessment is to determine whether the patient is competent to give his or her own history and what assistance might be needed to help ensure accuracy and precision of medical data. How is this informal assessment accomplished? First, certain clues about mental status arise even before the examination, as you observe the interaction between patient and family members or caretakers:

- Does the patient himself or herself call to make an appointment or to report symptoms?

- Does he or she arrive in the office alone, having driven a car or taken a bus or taxi?

- Does the patient forget an appointment even when reminded with a postcard or phone call?

Patients who cannot remember having made appointments may also be unable to remember medications, and, although these patients may experience symptoms, they may be unable to recall them and report them precisely to their physicians.

Next, as you enter the examining room or the patient's hospital room, you should pay careful attention to the patient's level of alertness (awake or drowsy). The patient sedated with a narcotic to alleviate renal colic may not be able to tell you very much (other than that he or she is feeling better now) until the medication wears off. Is the patient alert enough to focus attention on you and follow you from one question or statement to the next? Problems with alertness are common in hospitals and are probably underrecognized. You should also notice the patient's general appearance and behavior. Does he or she appear socially appropriate? Is the patient clean and quiet, or disheveled and agitated? Is the patient physically active or slow and retarded? As you begin the interview, you next assess the patient's verbal output or speech. Is it relevant or irrelevant? Rambling or reticent? Repetitious or almost mute? Coherent or incoherent? These characteristics, in turn, tell you a great deal about the patient's thought process and content. Is the pattern of thought logical or tangential? Is the patient preoccupied with thoughts of death? Does he or she have an obvious delusional system?

Here is an example of the opening moments of a follow-up visit with a 76-year-old woman who was brought in by her family because of weight loss and abdominal pain:

Dr: You said you've been feeling sad.

Pt: Yeah, my mother died before the baby was born, and I just started talking to the women about it and all of a sudden I said I couldn't. It's just sad. Well, I raised a boy, his name was Andy, and he stayed in Europe and he couldn't get out there and he was about 10 years or something like that. And then my sister, you know, wanted to come back and I went to look for the money we were trying to collect for. So I went up and—you know how it is—and on a Sunday I went over there and the baby was born.

How would you describe this patient's thought process? While her statement does seem vaguely related to the issue of sadness, it is difficult to follow the thread of this story, and it is certainly not a response to the question. We would describe it as rambling, tangential, and probably incoherent. It is typical of this patient, who could not really remember how she had been feeling. This is dementia, not psychosis.

In observing the patient, you will also certainly need to notice mood and affect. Is the patient flat or sad? Anxious or inappropriately merry? Cooperative or combative? Although orientation to time, place, and person may be obvious in the opening moments of your interview as you engage in social "chitchat" with your patient, be aware that many mildly and even moderately demented older persons retain excellent social skills that belie their cognitive deficit. We are reminded of two elderly women, both 93 years of age, who came to the office one day for back-to-back appointments. The nursing and reception staff commented, "Aren't they doing well!" But, in reality, one was doing well and the other was not. Each exhibited the social amenities of saying hello, observing how much she liked her doctor, and commenting on the weather. One then went on to give a detailed account of her arthritic symptoms over the past month; the other, despite enthusiastically greeting her doctor, whom she had seen many times before, replied as follows:

Pt: It's so very nice to see you. You're such a grand person.
Dr: Why, thank you. It's nice to see you, too. Do you remember who I am?
Pt: Well, you look very familiar. What's your name again?

The patient's ability to remember becomes readily apparent as the history proceeds and you try to gather precise information about symptoms. The elderly gentleman who repeats items in his history at different parts of a brief interview may not remember that he has already told you these details. The patient who says she has been feeling fine despite her family's concern about her repeated complaints of chest pain may not remember these episodes of pain. Indeed, sometimes you encounter obvious factual contradictions, such as a patient with surgical scars on her abdomen who states that she has never had surgery.

Formal Mental Status Testing

As summarized in the preceding paragraphs, much of the information required for formal mental status testing is readily obtainable during a careful medical interview. Usually, this is sufficient to assess your patient's reliability and rule out a significant organic mental problem such as delirium or dementia. Sometimes it is important to perform a more complete mental status evaluation that includes specific descriptions of the following:

- Appearance and behavior
- Attention and alertness
- Speech and language
- Mood and affect
- Memory and orientation
- Thought process and content
- Judgment and insight
- Abstract thinking, knowledge, and calculation

One semiquantitative tool that is often useful in this respect is the Mini-Mental Status Exam.[2] Although this questionnaire does not cover all the attributes of a complete mental status examination, it does give a relatively rapid and reliable numerical score estimating cognitive function. In the hospital, the Mini-Mental Status Exam can be used to follow patients with fluctuating mental status by administering it at various times, such as in the morning and evening. In the outpatient setting, it can be used to evaluate and follow patients who have problems with cognitive function over the course of months or years.

The Folstein Mini-Mental Status Exam is shown in Table 8–4. A score of 20 or greater is considered normal, whereas a score less than 20 suggests a neuropsychiatric or neurologic disorder such as delirium, dementia, or the pseudodementia of severe depression. Changing scores are also significant, even if they remain more than 20. For example, a patient who scores 30 in the morning and then 22 later that day definitely has a problem with cognition that demands the physician's attention. False-positive results may occur in patients who cannot concentrate because of extreme anxiety or thought disorder. In highly intelligent patients, the test may not be very sensitive, and, thus, false-negative results may occur. Such problems should be noted during the test; when in doubt, more complete cognitive testing (which is beyond the scope of this chapter) should be done.

Clinicians are often reluctant to do mental status testing and find it awkward to incorporate these tests into their interview format. Indeed, the data obtained are not really part of the medical history as such, but, more correctly, are part of the objective database, akin to the physical examination. Patients also may find specific questions about memory or cognition stressful. To ease these tensions, it is best to introduce mental status testing after the history part of your interaction, either just before or just after your physical examination. By this time, you will already have developed a relationship with your patient as well as an understanding of what some of his or her problems are. Such knowledge gives you a way to introduce this part of your evaluation in a straightforward and natural way. For example:

Dr: I've noticed that as we've been talking there are some things you have trouble remembering. Would it be all right if I test your memory?

Pt: How do you do that?

Dr: Well, I will ask you questions, some of which will seem silly to you and easy, and others may be hard for you. Would that be okay?

---

or

Dr: Do you ever forget to take your medication?

Pt: No, I never do.

Dr: How do you remember?

Pt: That's the first thing I do every day. But sometimes my memory is not so good. Sometimes I forget things I'm going to say.

Dr: Is that a new problem for you?

Pt: No, it has been for some time. I guess at 88, what can you expect?

Dr: At 88 I think you're doing fine. Would it be okay for me to test your memory so we can get an idea of how much of a problem it is?

TABLE 8–4 THE FOLSTEIN MINI-MENTAL STATUS EXAM

	Score	Maximum Score
Orientation		
What is the (year) _____ (season) _____ (month) _____ (date) _____ (day) _____?	( )	5
Where are we (state) _____ (county) _____ (town) _____ (hosp.) _____ (floor) _____?	( )	5
Registration		
I am going to name three objects and I want you to repeat them after me. (Interviewer, give one point for each correct answer. Repeat the objects until the patient can name them all—six trials maximum.) Number of trials ( ).	( )	3
Attention and Calculation		
I am going to ask you to do some subtraction. Think of the number 7. I want you to subtract 7 from 100. Now subtract 7 from that and keep on going. 100, _____, _____, _____, _____, _____. Stop. Alternative: Spell "world" backwards.	( )	5
Recall		
Please name the three objects that I had you repeat after me just a short while ago. (Interviewer, give one point for each correct answer.)	( )	3
Language		
Please name these for me. (Show patient a watch and a pencil.)	( )	2
Now, please repeat the following: "no ifs, ands, or buts."	( )	1
Now I am going to ask you to do something for me. "Take a paper in your right hand, fold it in half, and put it on the floor."	( )	3
Now I want you to read this and do what it says. (Interviewer, hand the patient a card that says "Close your eyes.")	( )	1
Now, please write a sentence for me on this blank piece of paper. (Interviewer, give the patient a blank piece of paper and ask him or her to write a sentence for you. Do not dictate a sentence; it must be written spontaneously. It must contain a subject and verb and be sensible. Correct grammar and punctuation are not necessary.)	( )	1
Visual-Motor Integrity		
Please copy this design. (Interviewer, on a clean piece of paper, draws intersecting pentagons, each side about 1 inch, and ask him or her to copy it exactly as it is. All 10 angles must be present and 2 must intersect to score 1 point.)	( )	1
TOTAL SCORE.	( )	30
INTERVIEWER: Assesses patient's level of consciousness along continuum.		

Alert	Drowsy	Stupor	Coma

SOURCE: From Folstein et al,[2] with permission. Pergamon Press PLC.

During the examination, patients will be more relaxed if you provide support and encouragement, especially when they struggle with finding the correct answers. For example:

Dr: Please name this for me. (Interviewer shows patient a pencil.)

Pt: Well, it's something for something to say in, I don't know.

Dr: Would you know how to use it?

Pt: No, I don't think so. I couldn't even write my name anymore.

Dr: You couldn't write your name anymore? Do you know what you could use this for?

Pt: I have no idea.

Dr: Okay, well it's a pencil.

Pt: A pencil.

Dr: You can write with it, you just do like this and you can write with it. I see that you wrote your name pretty well here.

Notice in this case how the physician provides information and positive reinforcement to the patient (an 82-year-old man with multi-infarct dementia) who, in fact, made a connection with the object ("I couldn't even write my name anymore") but was unable actually to name it or describe its use.

The Third Party

No discussion of interviewing elderly patients would be complete without mentioning the issue of autonomy and the role of concerned family members or caretakers. Difficulties arise when the patient and "concerned others" disagree on the extent of disability caused by dementia or other illness, or when the patient and family disagree about the value of some proposed plan of treatment. In the case of a failing or frail octogenarian with mild dementia, it is often difficult to evaluate competence for medical decision making or to assess the legitimate interests of family or caretakers. Within the interview, we may hear different histories: The family of an 80-year-old woman reports that she leaves the stove untended and soils herself, but the patient denies these problems. Family members may want to see the doctor in private, out of the patient's earshot; then they forbid the physician to discuss their concerns with the patient. Or a daughter brings her mother to the office pretty much against the patient's will. How do you respect the concerns of family members and at the same time nurture the patient's autonomy?

The preceding sentence contains two words that summarize the last paragraph (and indeed this entire section on interviewing elderly patients): respect and autonomy. First, you should approach your elderly patient with the same respect and concern that you have for any other patient. Your contract as a clinician includes honesty, privacy, and confidentiality, as discussed fully in Chapter 9. Consequently, while being sensitive to the family's concerns about what "grandma" should or should not be told about her condition, it is important for you to emphasize her right to know and the fact that most elderly patients respond well to being fully apprised of their situation. Moreover, be sensitive to the patient's feelings about privacy, and minimize the involvement of a third party in the interview if the patient so wishes. Respect for other family members demands that you make them aware at the outset of your clinician-patient contract: you will not collude with them to withhold information or to "help" the patient against his or her competent wishes.

Second, insofar as it is possible, nourish the patient's autonomy. Some elderly patients have deficits that render them temporarily or permanently incompetent to make medical decisions. However, even if your patient is judged incompetent, you continue to have an obligation to respect his or her interests. Sometimes you may disagree with family members about just what the patient's best interest *is*. For example, optimal medical treatment of an elderly, mildly demented man with heart disease might require a low-salt, cholesterol-lowering diet. This diet may eliminate most of the foods that he has enjoyed eating all his life. The patient's daughter might insist on sticking to "the letter of the law," cooking him only bland food that he doesn't like. Perhaps she believes this is in "Dad's best interest." "He doesn't know what's good for him," she tells the doctor. Doesn't he? It might be far more beneficial to the patient as a person to enjoy life and enjoy eating, than at age 75 years to have a small reduction in his cholesterol level. In this case, the clinician's obligation (nourishing autonomy) might be to counsel the daughter to provide a more enjoyable—though perhaps less medically "correct"—diet for her father.

S U M M A R Y : Techniques for Young and Old

Perhaps the theme common to interviewing patients at both ends of the age spectrum is the need to understand and respect the individual's ability—sometimes more and sometimes less—to engage in an autonomous and confidential doctor-patient relationship. Even the toddler can provide important data in the history, and most older persons do not require intermediaries, however well-meaning, to transmit their stories.

To make the most of your interactions with pediatric patients:

- Approach the young child indirectly by first admiring a toy or item of clothing.

- Understand the parent or guardian's view of the illness and re-assure them that they did not cause it.
- As the child gets older, clarify for both parent and child how the doctor-patient relationship becomes more confidential.
- Help families understand common problems and developmental milestones through the practice of anticipatory guidance.

To make the most of your interactions with geriatric patients:

- Adapt your interview style to a slower pace.
- Assess mental status through both informal observation and formal testing.
- Assess problems with activities of daily living.
- Do a detailed review of all medications, including over-the-counter medications.
- Respect the patient's life experience and nourish his or her autonomy.

With the ability to adapt your interview in both content and style to different age groups, you have begun the process of building on your basic skills and applying them to different situations and different types of patients. We continue this process as we move on to a discussion of more difficult interactions.

References

1. Duke University Center for the Study of Aging and Human Development. Multidimensional Functional Assessment: *The OARS Methodology*, 2nd Ed. Durham, NC: Duke University, 1978.
2. Folstein MF, Folstein SE, McHugh PR. Mini-mental state: A practical method for grading the cognitive state of patients for the clinician. *J Psychiatry Res* 1975; 12:189–198.

Suggested Readings

Bennett HJ. Using humor in the office setting: A pediatric perspective. *J Fam Pract* 1996; 42:462–464.

Steiner BD, Gest KL. Do adolescents want to hear preventive medicine counseling messages in outpatient settings? *J Fam Pract* 1996; 43:375–381.

CHAPTER 9

The Real Satisfaction

• • •

INTERACTING WITH THE PATIENT IN PRIMARY CARE

It's the humdrum, day-in, day-out, everyday work that is the real satisfaction of the practice of medicine; the million and a half patients a man has seen on his daily visits over a forty-year period of weekdays and Sundays that make up his life. I have never had a money practice; it would have been impossible for me.

William Carlos Williams, *The Autobiography*

Most medical care takes place in the clinician's office rather than in a hospital. Yet medical students have traditionally learned how to interview by doing "histories and physicals" on inpatients. In years past, the range of patients and illnesses seen in the hospital was reasonably broad and, because a person might have spent 2 weeks as an inpatient after an uncomplicated heart attack, or a week receiving IV antibiotics for pneumonia, it was convenient for students to spend an hour or more doing a "complete" history and physical. Such recovering patients often welcomed the students' company and attention. Today, hospitalized patients are usually both very ill and not particularly representative of the spectrum of clinical practice.

Learning to interview in the office setting presents its own set of problems. Normally, the clinician does not have an hour or more to spend with each patient, nor do patients necessarily expect to spend their day sitting in the physician's office; thus, efficiency and thoroughness may seem to conflict with one another. Because of its longitudinal nature, however, primary care practice presents many opportunities to use your interviewing skills to enhance patient care and develop effective physician-patient relationships. The first section of this chapter introduces various ways of improving physician-patient communication in the primary care setting. Subsequent sections consider additional issues in managed care, the importance of communication skills in avoiding malpractice suits, the clinical interview as a tool in preventive medicine, and the crucial role that confidentiality and truthfulness play in clinician-patient relationships.

SOLVING COMMUNICATION PROBLEMS IN PRIMARY CARE

Among the factors that sometimes lead to physician dissatisfaction in primary care are impairments in physician-patient communication. For example, Wendy Levinson and her coworkers[1] delineated six sources of frustration among practicing physicians in their relationships with patients:

- Lack of trust or agreement between physician and patient
- Patients with too many problems
- Physician feeling distressed in the encounter
- Lack of patient adherence
- Lack of understanding, patients who are too demanding or controlling
- Too many patients with difficult problems (e.g., substance abuse, chronic pain)

These situations are often the result of communication problems. Table 9–1 presents a short list of difficult interaction issues in primary care, presenting

TABLE 9–1 CAUSES OF FRUSTRATION IN PRIMARY CARE COMMUNICATION

Patient Perspective	Physician Perspective
The doctor doesn't listen to me.	I don't have enough time.
The doctor doesn't deal with all my problems.	The patient has too many problems.
The doctor doesn't explain anything.	The patient doesn't understand.
The doctor doesn't appreciate my suffering.	The patient brought this on himself.
The doctor makes me angry.	I dread this patient.

the patient's point of view as well as the physician's. In the following sections, we address each of these issues in turn and illustrate how good interviewing skills may convert sources of frustration into opportunities for better patient care.

The Doctor Doesn't Listen to Me/I Don't Have Enough Time

Sometimes a desire for efficiency tempts us to abandon an open-ended interviewing style in favor of more focused questioning; we think that if we ask just the right questions or follow an algorithm, we will save time. If the patient has chest pain, we will stick to chest pain questions; if he or she has an upset stomach, we will concentrate only on GI questions, and so forth. Another temptation is to cut the patient off before he or she finishes the opening statement, or perhaps even the chief complaint. It might be difficult to imagine a medical history without a chief complaint, but consider the following examples.

Example 1

Dr: Hello. You're here because of back pain?
Pt: Yes, I have lower back pain. And . . .
Dr: How long have you had it?

Example 2

Dr: Hi, how have you been? Let's see, I had you come back today to see how your depression is doing.
Pt: That part's okay. But . . .
Dr: How many pills are you up to now?

Example 3

Dr: How's it going?
Pt: Not too well, lot of discomfort here (puts his hand on back) down the arch and here under the arm and, ah, here, and this here . . . Remember, I keep complaining about that in the back . . .
Dr: How about the pacemaker clinic, were you there this morning?

Notice it is the physician, not the patient, who states the chief complaint in these examples. The physician has closed the inquiry to other problems or symptoms by indicating what topics he or she wants to discuss. In the third example, the physician completely ignores the patient's obvious back discomfort because he thinks of him as a cardiac patient. Beckman and Frankel[2] found in their study of internal medicine residents in an ambulatory clinic that the average time a patient was allowed to speak before being interrupted was only 18 seconds! Patients who are initially cut off are likely to be dissatisfied and try again and again to return to *their* concern; perhaps worse, they may simply give up and not have their problem addressed. How often the "heart" patient fails to have his arthritis evaluated because aching joints are not on the physician's agenda!

Paradoxically, you often save time by remaining quiet and allowing the patient to have his or her say. Open-ended questions allow you to generate hypotheses quickly without relying on the patient's hypotheses about his condition. Although questions such as, "How's your diabetes?" or "How's your chest pain?" also may sometimes be necessary, they should be delayed until later in the interview.

Here are some examples of better ways to begin with office patients:

Example 1

Dr: Hi, Mrs. Jones, I'm Dr. Walker. Nice to meet you.
Pt: Same here.
Dr: What brings you here today?
Pt: I'm having a problem with my back. It's still bothering me. And for the past 10 years, I've had a chronic problem with phlebitis in the legs, and I have some problem with my feet swelling at times and therefore circulation in both legs. But right now I'm having a devastating problem with my lower back. It's been going on ever since about the 20th of October. And I would like to see if I can get into a diet program.
Dr: A diet program?
Pt: Uh huh.
Dr: First, why don't you tell me about your back.

Example 2

Dr: What brings you here today?
Pt: Well, for several weeks now I've had these lumps on my head, they're really itchy . . . My neck hurts, too. I think it's from when I had that accident, you know, it keeps acting up. Since I am here, I might as well have it checked.
Dr: Okay. Have you had any other medical problems recently?

Example 3

Dr: Tell me why you came today.

Pt: Well, I haven't had physicals on a regular basis. I'm feeling like I'm getting to a point where I ought to do that.

Dr: So you need a good physical.

Pt: Right.

Dr: You sure it's not a specific problem you noticed?

Pt: Not really.

Dr: Okay. But if you think of something while we're talking, don't hesitate to mention it. How has your health been?

These physicians begin with open-ended questions that permit the patient to state a chief complaint and elaborate a bit on other concerns. In the third example, the physician notices the patient's apparent hedge ("Not really," as opposed to "No, not at all.") and reassures him that he is welcome to bring up symptoms as the interview progresses. In the second transcript, the physician listens to the patient's full response, then encourages additional disclosure, "Have you had any other medical problems recently?" Beckman and Frankel[2] found in their study that no completed statement of concerns required more than 150 seconds. These 2½ minutes (usually much less) may be the most critical time of the interview, avoiding frustration and anger on the part of both physician and patient and ensuring that the patient's "hidden" agenda does not *remain* hidden.

In ambulatory care, the patient's needs will dictate the character and completeness of your medical history at any given time. In one case, the history might be a database on a healthy person seeking guidance with regard to cardiac risk factors. In another situation, a patient may have an acute illness that demands immediate (and targeted) attention. Other primary care patients return for follow-up of chronic conditions that are influenced by medical, emotional, and social factors. Additionally, some chronically ill patients present with acute, perhaps unrelated, problems. Here is an example of a woman scheduled for a routine follow-up visit in an academic primary care center; she had developed a new symptom and some nonmedical concerns. The first-year family practice resident summarized the situation as follows (we have annotated the text to indicate the different types of problems):

> L.B. is a 50-year-old divorced woman whom I am seeing in follow-up for newly diagnosed diabetes mellitus and hypertension [chronic diseases]. She has been on glipizide, and her concerns for this visit are that about 1 week ago she experienced a dramatic change in her visual acuity [acute problem]. She states

that even with her glasses she is still unable to read as she had before. She can't see, her vision is blurry. She denies headaches or eye pain. She denies any other neurologic deficit. No numbness or tingling, no swelling of her extremities. Ms. B's other concern is that the Department of Labor states that if she has been ill she is unable to collect unemployment benefits [economic and social concern]. She requests a note stating that she is medically cleared to continue seeking work and, therefore, eligible for unemployment benefits. Her other problem is that she can't sleep because of anxiety, both about her job and also because of her former husband who keeps threatening her . . . [emotional and social concerns]

Given this complexity, you frequently cannot attend to all the issues in one visit. Fortunately, you do not have to. The complete database should evolve and develop, change and extend, over the course of your ongoing relationship with the patient.

The Doctor Doesn't Deal with All My Problems/The Patient Has Too Many Problems

What if the patient offers more complaints than you can handle in the time allotted? The solution begins with the opening moments of the encounter, during which you should not only demonstrate openness but also set the agenda for this visit. When the patient presents several concerns, you must establish priorities. What has to be attended to today? Next week? Next month? What problem is of most concern to the patient? To the physician? When there is disagreement between doctor and patient about these priorities, it is the physician's responsibility to take the lead in negotiating a resolution of the "conflict" (see Chap. 15). Table 9–2 summarizes various techniques that will help you to avoid the "doorknob phenomenon," in which

TABLE 9–2   THE SATISFACTORY ENCOUNTER: HOW TO AVOID THE "HAND-ON-THE-DOORKNOB PHENOMENON"

From the Beginning of the Encounter:	In Transition to Closing the Encounter:
• Orient the patient to the flow of the visit.	• Orient the patient to closure.
• Set priorities: What needs to be done today?	• Summarize the visit.
	• Check for patient understanding.
• Address emotions and psychosocial issues.	• Clarify the plan.
• Explore patient beliefs and expectations.	• Encourage and reassure the patient.
• Provide opportunities for questions.	

*Adapted from White, Levinson, and Roter.[3]

the patient presents new concerns (sometimes the most pressing problem of all!) as you are about to leave the room. For example, as you escort the patient to the door, he or she says, "By the way, I have this crushing substernal chest pain." What do you say at that point? Unrevealed agendas lead to missed diagnoses (some of them life-threatening), not to mention angry patients (who feel that they did not get what they came for; see Table 9–1) and frustrated physicians (who get telephone calls later the same day from patients who have just left the office and now have "new" complaints).

After the patient's opening statement, the physician should encourage the patient to "lay the cards on the table" by specifying all of today's concerns. This initial phase establishes the range of problems and their breadth, but not their depth. It may be likened to the overture of a musical score in which each theme is briefly introduced but then dropped, only to be developed more fully later. In music, certain conventions and the composer's artistry determine the order in which the themes or melodies may be developed; in medical interviewing, the clinician and the patient decide how to proceed. When one problem is not clearly more urgent than another, the patient may be the one to decide how to use the limited time. However, when there is an urgent problem that the patient does not recognize, or if the patient is not capable of making decisions, the physician must play a more direct role in setting the agenda.

When there is more than one problem and none is clearly more urgent than another, a summary statement followed by a question and an explanation of your strategy may help:

- "You've mentioned three concerns—your weight, this pain in your foot, and the premenstrual symptoms. Since our time is limited, which one would you like to focus on today (or first)?"

- "I can see that you're really bothered by this itching in your feet (summary statement and interchangeable response). But I noticed that your weight is up about 10 pounds and you seem a little short of breath. Since our time is limited, is it okay if we check out your heart and lungs first?"

It is easy to overlook new problems when a patient is scheduled for what looks like a routine follow-up visit and you start the interview off with, "How's the diabetes doing?" as opposed to, "How have things been going lately?" The latter is totally unrestricted and may even invite nonmedical responses like, "My health is great, but my job is driving me crazy." "How has your health been?" or "How have your medical problems been doing?" are intermediate queries restricted to whatever concerns the patient perceives as health-related. "What can I do for you today?" is a good beginning; it is open-ended yet indicates the desire to focus on "today."

Here is an example of how you might begin an interim history for a patient with a number of chronic health problems:

Dr: Tell me why you came in today.

Pt: Just my regular visit. Dr. Smith said I had to come back for a checkup.

Dr: A checkup?

Pt: Yeah, he said I needed to have my blood sugar rechecked after he changed the medication.

Dr: Okay, fine. We can certainly take care of that. Anything else I should know about or that we should discuss before we get to that? Are you having any other problems?

Pt: Well, since my last visit I've noticed some trouble with my breathing.

Notice how the physician makes sure nothing else is going on. The blood sugar may not be an immediate priority if the patient has developed shortness of breath, possibly suggesting congestive heart failure. This search for other active problems (OAPs, see Chap. 4) is an essential part of every initial or follow-up outpatient interview. In contrast to the initial interview of a hospitalized patient, where the discussion of OAPs tends to occur after the complete development of the history of the present illness, in the ambulatory setting, particularly for those with chronic disease, the discussion of OAPs occurs early. The search for OAPs is essential in setting the agenda to make the most efficient use of your brief time with the patient. In this context, the OAPs pretty much replace the complete ROS, which neither the physician nor the patient has the tolerance to repeat on each and every visit.

We close this section with one final example. This is the opening segment of an interview with a 60-year-old woman who scheduled an appointment because she had been having chest pain. Notice the physician's confusion as she states her chief complaint:

Dr: How are you feeling today?

Pt: Oh, not too good. I still have that goofy headache.

Dr: You still have the headache?

Pt: And it's, I would say, one side, just sick. It's on the right side, and it starts here and it goes to the top of my head.

Dr: Have you ever had a headache like this before?

Pt: Oh, I've had headaches ever since 1950. I would take attacks and my blood pressure was very high and the doctor gave me medication.

Dr: I see. Is there anything different about this headache that you have right now compared to your other headaches that you've had?

Pt: Compared to the other headaches, this one is not quite as bad. But I've had it several days and it started about Sunday, and I'm worried about my blood pressure. Then I started having those chest pains.

Dr: And you've been having chest pains? Tell me about them. (search for OAPs)

Pt: Well, they're right here. (Patient points to right pectoral area and then reaches around to her back.) It's right up in here and down around in there. Sharp. Like I went to pick up something off the dresser and it just grabbed me.

Dr: Okay. And you're also worried about your pressure? (OAPs)

Pt: When I went to the store, I took it on the machine. It was a hundred and ninety something.

Dr: Okay. What would you say is the thing that's worrying you the most right now?

Notice that the physician has established both the range of problems (at least three) as well as their urgency (none seems particularly urgent—the headaches are old and no worse, the chest pain is probably musculoskeletal, and the blood pressure has been taken in the office and is 140/90). Given the limited time available, the physician now turns the agenda over to the patient, who will dictate which concern to deal with during this encounter. (By the way, this is the patient we met in Chapter 5, who actually answered the physician's last question by saying her main worry was "how to get those bills paid." So the agenda in this case was, indeed, completely hidden until the clinician permitted the patient to decide how best to use the visit.)

The Doctor Doesn't Explain Anything/The Patient Doesn't Understand

Studies repeatedly show that medical treatment is "taken as directed" in only 50 percent or less of cases; understanding is one of the most important factors in patient adherence to therapy. We prefer not to use the term "non-compliance" (see Chap. 15) because it evokes the image of a passive, irresponsible patient behaving like a child; in fact, patients often have very good reasons not to follow their physicians' instructions. Nonetheless, medical treatment is often compromised because the patient simply does not understand the nature and severity of his or her illness or the nature of prescribed medication, the expected outcome of treatment, and the specific directions for taking it.

Presuming that physicians attempt to explain these issues to their patients, why don't patients remember what their physicians tell them? Investigators have shown that personal characteristics, such as age and intelligence, generally do not play a major role in how much is remembered.

Likewise, the obvious method of writing down the information, which on the surface would appear to be a fail-safe method, does not necessarily lead to better recall of information.

Patients will be more satisfied with their care and will follow instructions better if they remember what the doctor tells them. Here is an example of the final part of a diagnostic interview in which, among other problems, the doctor appears to pay little attention to conveying understandable information in the communication:

Dr: Okay, Mr. H, you've been having these problems for some time and I think they warrant further investigation. I'm not quite sure right now, some of your symptoms seem to be upper GI but some seem to be colonic as well. It could be an ulcer problem, it could be inflammatory bowel disease. I think the first thing to do is to schedule a flexible sigmoidoscopy and then we'll go on from there. I can do the flex sig in the office here later on this week. The nurse can give you an exact time and meanwhile we'll get you scheduled on the x-rays. You'll need a barium enema, probably air contrast, and then an upper GI series . . .

Pt: Is that test you mentioned, is that where you insert a tube in my rectum? I had one of those about 2 years ago, I could hardly stand it.

Dr: Well, it's not the most comfortable thing, but it is important—it's the only way you can get to the rectum, look at it, see the problem. It's not as bad as you think.

Pt: The main problem I'm having is this bloated feeling, and the indigestion. I didn't think it was so serious. Isn't there some medicine?

Dr: As you said, it's been bothering you for quite some time, so I think we ought to get to the bottom of it. You can never be too careful. The problem with the GI tract is that, a lot of times, symptoms seem to blend together and it's hard to know what you're dealing with unless you look.

Pt: Do you think it might be something serious, I mean like an ulcer or something . . .

Dr: Well, it could be an ulcer, but it's not typical. I think we'll just have to do the work-up and see. In the meantime, I'm going to give you an antispasmodic drug to take, you can take it with every meal and at bedtime. I'll give you a prescription. We'll see what happens.

Let us focus first on the doctor's initial statement in this transcript. How might this physician have presented the information in such a way as to facilitate understanding? First, the physician could have used words and phrases more likely to be understood by the patient. The terms "inflammatory bowel disease" and "flexible sigmoidoscopy" should not have been employed unless the doctor intended to explain them, or at least check with the patient to determine whether he knows what they mean. Medical jargon can creep into any conversation. Anything important to the patient that goes on in his or her body can be described in plain language. (Often, the difficulty in translation results from our own failure to have fully mastered a particular concept.)

Second, the physician in the example could have been concrete and specific about the problems being considered, the steps in the diagnostic plan, and the benefits and risks of his approach. On the contrary, the physician spoke in abstract and general terms like "further investigation" and "go on from there." What does that mean? This physician was uncertain about the precise diagnosis, but nonetheless he could have been more concrete and explicit about what the options were and, more importantly for the patient's peace of mind, what the likely outcome would be: Will I get better? Is my condition serious? Is it likely that I'll need surgery? Eric Cassell coined the term "vague reference" to characterize this technique of tangential communication with patients that often leads to increased, rather than decreased, anxiety about the problem because it encourages the patient to imagine the worst.

Third, the physician in our example could have stated the most important information concisely at the beginning. Patients are more likely to remember the initial chunk of information than data presented later in a discussion. You should hook the patient's memory by giving a succinct statement that puts the problem in a frame of reference and leads to "here's how we'll deal with it." The clinician might then use another technique, repetition, to bring home the salient points during subsequent discussion with the patient.

Last, at the end of the segment, the physician could have inquired about how much the patient understood and given him some feedback about that understanding. The clinician could also have encouraged questions. Note that these techniques for maximizing patient education also help avoid the "doorknob phenomenon" (see previous section). The simple technique of asking the patient to repeat what you have said and then giving feedback substantially increases patient satisfaction while increasing accurate recall of information.

Taking the example as a whole, notice that the clinician is attempting to share his uncertainty with the patient. The clinical situation is truly ambiguous and the physician's statements accurately convey that fact. However, the manner in which he conveys the ambiguity is neither educational nor anxiety-reducing. In fact, it creates new questions while leaving the old one ("Is it something serious?") unanswered. Moreover, the physician has really not given any advice to the patient about his problem. While the diagnosis is admittedly unclear, the physician does have considerably more knowledge about what the symptoms mean and what might be done about them than the patient has. The physician could have used this opportunity to decrease some of the patient's uncertainty while mobilizing his efforts to address the problem constructively. For example, here is how the same clinician might, on a better day, share his findings and arrive at a plan with the patient:

Dr: Well, Mr. H, you've had a difficult time with this problem, but I believe we'll be able to get to the bottom of it and find out what's wrong. We will have to do some additional tests, though, before we can say for sure. Your main symptoms—the cramps you get and the loose bowels—are most likely caused by a problem in your colon, one that we call irritable bowel syndrome. That means that there's a spasm in the muscles of your large bowel, and that gives you the cramps and so on. But your other symptoms, that bloated feeling in the stomach and pain up there, they also suggest an acid problem, like ulcer or gastritis.

Pt: Are any of those serious?

Dr: They're all medical problems that can be treated or cured. There's nothing to suggest that you have something really serious like cancer, for example. It could be an ulcer, but I think it's more likely that irritable bowel syndrome can explain all of your symptoms.

Pt: I really want to get to the bottom of this, I just can't take it anymore. I just can't get my work done feeling like I do now.

Dr: It sounds like these attacks have really gotten to you . . .

Pt: I'd say I'm almost paralyzed.

Dr: Okay, I understand. What I'd like to do is to schedule some tests today. One of them is a flexible sigmoidoscopy; that's a procedure in which I insert a flexible tube into your rectum. I can look through it and check the lining of your bowel, like for irritation or hemorrhoids. You'll come back to my office for that. The other two tests are x-rays, one of the large bowel and one of the stomach and small bowel.

Pt: Do you think it might be something serious, like an ulcer or something?

Dr: What are you thinking about? Possibly it could be an ulcer . . .

Pt: Well, ulcers can kill you, can't they?

Dr: It sounds like you heard something bad about ulcers.

Pt: My uncle bled to death from one. First they said it was an ulcer, then it didn't heal—he couldn't eat anything. Finally they found out it was cancer.

Dr: And you're worried that this could be cancer, even if the tests show something else?

Pt: I don't know. Like I say, I can't take it anymore. My nerves are part of it, maybe.

Dr: Let's take this a step at a time. First, your symptoms and my examination do not show any suggestion of cancer; we have no reason to suspect it. As I said, it really sounds like either an acid problem or irritable bowel. That's the most likely. Let me explain that a little more. . . .

This time the physician has used a number of techniques that will help enhance patient understanding and cooperation (Table 9–3). The patient is likely to be more satisfied than in our first example and to go home less anxious about his condition. In addition, the doctor also actively elicited the patient's beliefs ("It sounds like you heard something bad . . . ") and took them into account in his explanation. We discuss patients' health beliefs and expectations in Chapter 14.

The Doctor Doesn't Appreciate My Suffering/The Patient Brought This on Himself or Herself

With so much emphasis these days on the impact of lifestyle on health and illness, it is common to see patients who appear "responsible" for their disease states. The patient who smokes and develops chronic lung disease (and still refuses to quit) or who continues to eat improperly despite obesity, hyperlipidemia, and diabetes, seems, perhaps, deserving of the consequences of his or her actions, whether such consequences be the additional suffering brought about by lung cancer or the development of severe degenerative joint disease with unremitting pain. When such patients, unable to change, still expect our support in relieving their pain and suffering (what audacity!), it is all too easy for us to blame them for their sorry state, and thereby absolve ourselves of the helper/healer role. What is worse, our usual sympathy may be quickly exhausted in what seems a never-ending cycle of trying to help patients we think should help themselves; in our frustration we may display negative and even punitive feelings toward these patients. These feelings are explored in detail in Chapter 10.

TABLE 9–3 MAXIMIZING PATIENT UNDERSTANDING

Use plain English rather than medical jargon.

Use concrete and specific language; avoid vague references.

State the important message first; then use repetition to reinforce it.

Ask the patient to restate the message.

Give corrective feedback.

Provide opportunities for questions.

The Doctor Makes Me Angry/I Dread This Patient

Perhaps a more disturbing problem among clinicians with long-term relationships with patients is that they occasionally see patients who actually make them feel distressed during the encounter (and sometimes long after). This distress may be experienced as a sinking feeling in the pit of one's stomach at the sight of a certain individual's chart on the "call-back" pile, or the sight of the patient's name on a full appointment schedule. Or the distress may be more overt—a conscious wish for the patient to seek care elsewhere. It is confusing for us in our helper/healer role to see patients become angry with us and to find ourselves, in turn, rejecting the patient. Sorting out what these patients are angry about is not easy. Is it their terminal illness? Is it their depression, which makes them irritable and seemingly angry at everything, including us? Is it our office, which malfunctions and fails to meet their needs? Or is it something that we either omit or commit in the physician-patient relationship that causes tension and, occasionally, downright antagonism? To further confuse matters, what looks like anger at us may well be something else entirely—frustration on the job or in a marital relationship, for instance—that spills over into the doctor's office. These issues, as well as skills to help you identify the source of such feelings and overcome them, are also dealt with at length in Chapter 10.

SPECIFIC ISSUES IN MANAGED-CARE SETTINGS

Managed-care practices are rapidly becoming the norm, rather than the exception, in American medical practice. These arrangements are characterized by the fact that insurers "manage" the services available to a given patient by offering comprehensive systems of care that range from preventive services and primary care through subspecialty and tertiary care. Among their more attractive features, managed-care programs require each person to identify a participating primary care physician, who will then coordinate the patient's total health care. Another attractive feature is the frequent emphasis on prevention, including behavioral-change programs (e.g., smoking cessation, weight loss).

The more troublesome features of managed care arise not so much from the concept itself but from its current implementation. Because health insurance in the United States is overwhelmingly employer-based, people tend to change their insurance when they change jobs. Moreover, in today's competitive environment, several plans may compete annually for a given employer's contract. Thus, an employee's health insurance may change frequently, requiring him or her to change primary care physicians each time. A second troublesome problem arises from the "dark side" of making the primary care provider integral to the system. Because many patients are accustomed to dealing with several different specialist physicians, the requirement to obtain referrals for each from a primary care physician may be perceived by them as burdensome. Moreover, when the generalist physician attempts to provide more rational care by limiting the fragmentation of services, thereby acting as the patient's advocate, some patients believe the physician is acting as a gatekeeper to prevent access to a desired service. This conflict in beliefs and expectations may fuel dissatisfaction among both patients and physicians.

Because these two managed-care problems—the need to change clinicians and a conflict in agendas—are general issues in clinician-patient interactions and not limited to certain settings, we consider them as additional primary care issues.

"Coerced" Change

Consider this opening exchange between a patient and her new physician at MagnaCare, a managed-care program:

Dr: What can I do for you, Ms. B?

Pt: Well, they told me I had to come in and see you. What happened is, my health insurance changed and now I can't see my regular doctor anymore . . . I've been going to him for about 10 years now. He knows my whole history, everything . . .

This physician has a serious handicap: the patient seems upset that she can't see her "regular" doctor and has only come because "they" told her to. The patient's opening statement is not, in fact, about what the symptoms are, but about the patient's frustration and possible anger. The temptation here is for the physician to ignore or minimize the patient's concerns and try to get on immediately with the chief complaint, perhaps by saying, "Okay, but tell me what your medical problem is," or "That's too bad, but we can get copies of his records. . . . Now what is your problem today?" The second statement acknowledges the situation but fails to consider the patient's feelings. It seems to imply that the medical record captures everything that's important in a physician-patient relationship; people are interchangeable.

How might this physician respond in a more effective way? Consider the following two statements:

Response 1

Dr: (after a few seconds pause) It sounds like you had a good relationship with your doctor.

Response 2

> **Dr:** It must be really frustrating when that happens. You probably just picked my name out of the book and you don't know what to expect.

In both cases the physician gives an empathic, interchangeable response (see p. 29). In the first case, he demonstrates an understanding of the cognitive content (previous relationship); in the second, he focuses on affective content (frustration). Both of these are appropriate in this situation. The second response goes a bit further in that it addresses an additional area of concern: the patient's uncertainty of what to expect from a new physician. It gives the patient permission to verbalize her fears. For example, the conversation might continue:

> **Pt:** Well, yes, I just had to go through the MagnaCare list, so I tried you because it's pretty convenient to get to your office. My regular doctor was Dr. Samuels, just up the road in Port Jefferson. He's been treating me for years for my diabetes and arthritis.
>
> **Dr:** Oh, I know Dr. Samuels. He's a good internist. I understand why you hate to be forced to leave him. Well, I'll try to do a good job for you too. And we can send for a copy of your records at Dr. Samuels' office.

This vignette of "coerced" change serves as an example of the general rules to begin listening at the beginning and to attempt to remove barriers to effective communication as soon as you identify them.

Dueling Agendas

> **Dr:** How can I help you, Mr. C?
>
> **Pt:** They told me I had to see my PCP (primary care provider) to get these referrals (brings out a list). I have an appointment next Tuesday with Dr. Nephron, who treats me for blood pressure, so I need that one today. And then my regular follow-ups with my allergist, my diabetes specialist— by the way, my sugar's high—and my cardiologist are due. So I thought I'd better get those referrals now, so I don't have to keep calling your office. And while I'm here, I was also wondering if you could recommend a good specialist for my stomach.

How would you feel if you were this patient's primary care physician? The patient is acting as if the physician were a clerk or a gatekeeper; from his perspective, the physician's sole function is to handle the paperwork to enable him to see an array of specialist physicians. This PCP—to use today's managed-care jargon—is bound to feel unappreciated and, perhaps, angry. The PCP might be tempted to reply: "Wait a second, that's not how things work here. I'm the one who decides what referrals you need!" This would almost certainly lead to a needless confrontation. The problem, of course, is that the patient and physician here have radically different agendas: the physician sees himself as taking care of the patient and addressing his illness; the patient views the doctor as an administrative cog.

Dueling agendas demand a direct approach. Unlike the "coerced change" example, it is unlikely that simple facilitative responses will encourage the patient to accept the physician's care. The issue here is a radical misunderstanding of (or disagreement with) the role of the PCP in general and, more specifically, in the managed-care scheme. If the physician tried a simple interchangeable response like, "Well, Mr. C, it sounds like you have quite a few medical problems," the patient is likely to agree and indicate that that is precisely why he needs so many doctors. What is required here is a clear and relatively complete educational statement, such as:

Dr: Well, Mr. C, it sounds like you've needed quite a few specialists, and certainly if you have an appointment with Dr. Nephron on Tuesday, I agree that we should arrange a referral for you . . . But today we're scheduled for a new-patient visit—that means a complete check-up—so I think we should get started so I can understand your problems better. Did you have a primary care doctor before you joined MagnaCare?

Pt: Not really. I used to go to Dr. Smith for colds and things, you know, maybe once a year, but he never did any testing . . . just wrote me a prescription for antibiotics or something.

Dr: OK, then, let me start by explaining how I view my role. I'd like to be your main doctor and coordinate all your medical care. And I'd like get to know you a little better, so that maybe together we can work on improving your health. If we decide that you need to see a specialist, then he'll report back to me and we can talk about it. Now I don't think we can start out with all these referrals . . . first, I need to understand your health problems. So I suggest we start from what's bothering you right now—your stomach—and then we can talk about your sugar and your heart and so forth. How's that?"

Pt: Well OK, but it's a long story . . .

This, of course, is not a miraculous resolution to dueling agendas; there will probably be continued tension over referrals, requiring additional education and, possibly, confrontation. Note, however, four aspects of this physician's approach. First, he immediately acknowledges the patient's most pressing request: the appointment with Dr. Nephron. Whether or not a nephrologist is required, the PCP minimizes the disruption to the patient's style by acceding to that referral. Presumably, he decided the referral would buy him some time to establish a relationship based on education and negotiation. Second, the PCP immediately begins to establish the ground rules, including the fact that he views himself as the patient's major care provider. The message to Mr. C is clear, although not fully detailed as yet. Third, he states his case without reference to MagnaCare rules or expectations; good medical care should be justified on its own merits. Had the physician said, "You're in MagnaCare now, so let me explain the restrictions they have on referrals to specialists . . . ," he would, to some extent, be opting out of his therapeutic role by engaging in a game of "us versus them." Finally, the PCP is reasonable and friendly in his explanation; though he speaks firmly, he has not yielded to the understandable impulse to begin with, "What do you think this is, a supermarket where you can come in and pick out anything you want?"

Although dueling agendas may at times be a particularly acute problem in managed care arrangements, this dynamic is important throughout primary care and, indeed, in all forms of clinical practice. We present additional examples in the section on "Papers, Forms, and Clearances" (p. 178) and consider the subject in more detail in Chapter 15.

PREVENTIVE HEALTH CARE

Preventive health services are an extremely important part of primary care. Good physician-patient communication plays a central role in prevention. The medical interview allows you to identify the patient's risk-related behaviors, personal preferences, and needed preventive services; interviewing skills also facilitate health education, negotiation, and counseling regarding healthy lifestyles. In these ways the medical interview can be a powerful tool for promoting better health. Table 9–4 outlines the components of a pre-

TABLE 9–4   THE PREVENTIVE HEALTH ASSESSMENT

Immunization Status	Specific Risk Factors
Recommended vaccines	Behaviors
Are they up to date?	Exposures
Screening	Clinical findings
Recommended tests	Healthy Lifestyles
Are they up to date?	Behaviors
Family History	Beliefs
Diseases and disorders	

ventive care assessment. Normally, of course, these features should be embedded in the initial medical interview.

Unfortunately, immunizations and early detection (screening tests) are frequently neglected in ambulatory medicine because office visits are commonly short and highly focused. In these circumstances, physicians may forget to build a database regarding a patient's immunization status and appropriate screening tests. Thus, it is important to include such questions as part of the past medical history during the initial interview; subsequently, they should form a prominent part of a patient's annual check-up. It is helpful to begin a segment about prevention and screening tests with a brief introduction, such as: "Now I'd like to ask a few questions about preventive care."

As part of the initial medical history, the patient profile should provide you with information about major cardiovascular and cancer risk factors—cigarette smoking, dietary preferences, exercise habits, occupational exposures, alcohol and other drug use. Additional risk factors may be identified in the past medical history (e.g., history of hypertension, diabetes, or elevated cholesterol), and family history (e.g., father had a first heart attack at an early age, or mother died of breast cancer).

CONFIDENTIALITY AND TRUTHFULNESS

Maintaining Confidentiality

Confidentiality is an ancient concept in medicine. The Hippocratic Oath states, "What I may see or hear in the course of the treatment or even outside of the treatment in regard to the life of men, which on no account one must spread abroad, I will keep to myself holding such things shameful to be spoken about."[4] The American Medical Association's Principles of Ethics state that "a physician . . . shall safeguard patient confidences within the constraints of the law." The ethical principle of respect for persons dictates a right to privacy that would be violated if we were to make personal information available to others. Likewise, confidentiality facilitates openness of communication and a trusting relationship between patient and physician, thereby enhancing therapeutic effectiveness.

How do we maintain confidentiality as clinicians in a modern medical practice? First, we need to develop the habit of discretion. Confidentiality does not simply mean keeping an occasional big secret but rather indicates a daily pattern of respect for patients and their stories. This means that discussion of cases with friends, roommates, or spouses is generally inappropriate, even when the information in question is not strictly personal. Of course, some people do have a right to know. Medicine is a collegial enterprise. Clinicians function as members of teams; consequently, we often need to discuss patients with our peers, consultants, and other health-care professionals. As learners, we have a particular obligation to discuss patients with our teachers; even here, however, discretion is important. There is rarely any justification for talking about patients on crowded elevators or in other public settings. In the hospital, presenting patients at the bedside is often a good teaching technique, but it may infringe on confidentiality if a roommate can hear the patient's personal life being discussed.

Another important way of maintaining confidentiality is to write only appropriate information in the patient's clinical record (see Chap. 7, p. 122). You should approach the record as a document that the patient could review at any time. Especially with regard to sensitive information, you should always ask yourself whether writing a particular item in the chart is important to your patient's care. Some examples of sensitive information include details of sexual practices, a criminal record, marital conflict, and financial difficulties. Mental illness, suicide attempts, and substance abuse are also topics that, although they must be recorded, should be handled sensitively. In some cases it might be possible to write a brief "neutral" note to jog your memory, without expressing lurid details. Psychiatrists often keep their records in a personal file separate from the general medical record as a method of maximizing confidentiality while minimizing access.

Limits and Exceptions

Confidentiality is a qualified duty, not an absolute one. Table 9–5 presents some standard exceptions to the rule of confidentiality. If a patient develops a seizure disorder, for example, a physician might be required by law to report this fact to the state agency that issues driver's licenses. This might lead to the license being suspended until the patient is medically stable and certified "seizure free" for a specified period of time. Such laws are intended to prevent automobile accidents, but they may cause hardship for individuals who, for example, need to drive to work. Similarly, reporting suspected child abuse or domestic violence can cause a great deal of short-term family disruption and suffering, but the physician must do so if he or she judges abuse to be probable; the physician is supported by law because the state has in-

TABLE 9–5 JUSTIFIED EXCEPTIONS TO CONFIDENTIALITY

Required by Law*	Threats of Harm to Patient or Others
Gunshot wounds	Death threats
Specified communicable diseases	Suicidality
Child abuse or neglect	Communicable diseases
Dog bites	
Licensing requirements (e.g., drivers, pilots)	
Court subpoenas	

*These are examples; specific requirements differ by jurisdiction.

tervened to protect the interests of vulnerable persons who cannot protect themselves.

Although clinicians must always strive to maintain confidentiality, they should also be aware of the increasing difficulty in doing so and the growing tension between the dictates of privacy and demands of interested third parties. These problems result from:

- New health-care arrangements in which the physician is actually employed by a third party (e.g., health maintenance organization, managed-care company, or corporate medical department) and may, therefore, have obligations other than those to his or her patients

- The use of broad, open-ended release forms to obtain medical information to judge disability, insurability, and employability

- Computerized medical information systems to which large numbers of people might have access

These forces highlight the need to explain to patients that there may be situations in which you are obliged to share information. When such a situation arises, notify the patient and attempt to secure his or her permission. Failing that, be truthful about what is required and what you intend to do. If you diagnose a case of, for example, syphilis or tuberculosis, explain that the law dictates that you must submit a report to the health department. While describing the public health reasons for this report, you are also giving the patient crucial information about communicability and its implications for his or her behavior.

Papers, Forms, and Clearances: Questions About Truthfulness

Bureaucratic paperwork is the bane of modern medical practice. Enormous numbers of patient-physician encounters are generated because people must have medical forms completed for jobs, school, insurance, public assistance, nursing homes, social programs, driver's licenses, and so forth. Likewise, health insurers require the proper paperwork to justify payment for medical or laboratory services. Managed-care organizations often require primary-care physicians to fill out forms for each specialist referral—sometimes for each visit. It is understandable that physicians are not inclined to devote their best clinical judgment or their finest literary efforts to grinding out such administrative fodder. However, truthfulness in everyday medical practice requires honesty in the way we handle these bureaucratic headaches.

Two issues frequently arise with regard to clearances and certifications in primary care. In one case, the patient asks that information be suppressed:

- Pt: Don't put down that I'm a diabetic. After all, my diabetes is in good control. And it'll cost me plenty in extra insurance premiums.

- Pt: Listen, that nervous breakdown was 3 years ago. It won't happen again. I'm all right now.

What should you do, given the fact that telling the truth might well result in significant adverse consequences for your patient?

First, be honest in answering explicit questions on the form. You should explain this to the patient beforehand so he or she does not have false expectations when giving consent for you to share medical information.

Second, take the time to write additional explanatory material if you believe that it will benefit the patient. You might indicate that the hypertension or diabetes is in excellent control or that the episode of depression has completely resolved with no residual symptoms.

Finally, don't volunteer information unless you have reason to believe it is relevant. Often, a final question will ask something like, "Any other significant medical problems or conditions?" There is no need here to detail the patient's medical history; simply put what might, in your clinical judgment, be significant to the insurance or job or program in question.

A different problem arises when patients ask you to make false or unsupported assertions about their illness or disability. The patient's insurance carrier or the state welfare department might ask if, in your opinion, the patient is "totally disabled." Perhaps you are unable to ascertain objective evidence of disability, or the evidence is quite limited. "Yes, Mr. X does have diabetes, but there are only minor symptoms and no long-term sequelae." Or, "Yes, Mrs. Y does have degenerative joint disease but this, in my opinion, cannot explain her chronic pain." (Of course, chronic pain is in itself a severe disability, whether or not an "objective" cause can be identified.) The important issue here is that you should never make assessments of disability that are not warranted by your clinical judgment; be truthful in your medical assessment. You can, of course, refuse to complete a form if you feel that your opinion is not in the patient's best interest.

MALPRACTICE LIABILITY

A few years ago, the issue of malpractice liability would not have been mentioned in a textbook on clinical interviewing skills, especially in a chapter dealing with interactions in primary care. Physicians then thought (as many still do) that the best way to avoid being sued was to practice so-called defensive medicine; that is, to engage in a pattern of practice in which one makes medical decisions based on perceived liability, rather than on good clinical judgment. The emergency medicine physician might, for example, routinely order CT scans on patients with head injuries, even if clinical circumstances do not warrant the scan. Similarly, the internist or neurologist might order an MRI on all patients with headache, knowing, of course, that the vast majority of such scans are not clinically indicated. Since that time, studies of malpractice claims have repeatedly demonstrated two remarkable findings:

- *Defensive medicine **does not** prevent malpractice suits.* If a patient has a bad medical outcome, the fact that his physician ordered extra (and inappropriate) tests does not reduce the risk of the physician being sued. The best policy, in fact, is to follow clinical guidelines or the standard of care.

- Good *physician-patient communication* **does** *prevent malpractice suits.* A patient who feels that the physician listens to and understands him or her is not likely to sue that physician, even if the treatment has a bad outcome.[5-7]

Good physician-patient interaction is, in fact, the best defensive medicine. Because this finding is so consistent and striking, malpractice insurance carriers have begun to sponsor communication skills seminars for physicians. Physicians who complete these seminars often receive discounts on their malpractice insurance premiums. An empathic, compassionate approach with good interactive techniques leads to better diagnosis and therapy. This approach also enhances patient satisfaction. Satisfied patients generally do not sue their physicians. In fact, if an adverse outcome of care occurs, the strongest predictor of a malpractice action being brought against the physician is a pre-existing poor physician-patient relationship.[5-7]

These findings have several implications for primary care, as well as all other aspects of medical practice. In particular, to minimize your risk of being sued:

- Develop and nourish the therapeutic core qualities of empathy, respect, and genuineness (Chap. 2)
- Focus on the interview as your main diagnostic tool: the more you listen, the more you will learn (Chaps. 3 through 6)
- Develop good clinical judgment (Chap. 13)
- Enhance communication skills that facilitate effective physician–patient relationships (this chapter and Chaps. 14 and 15)

S U M M A R Y : Communication in Primary Care Practice

Primary-care practice can be the source of great satisfaction in medicine. In some cases, though, problems in clinician-patient communication lead to dissatisfaction of both patients and physicians. Managed-care arrangements can exacerbate some of these interactive concerns and present new ones. In this chapter we reviewed several such problems and suggested skills to help address them:

- No time to listen? Allow the patient time to state his or her concerns.
- Too many problems? Set the agenda.

- The patient doesn't understand? Explain the issues in plain language and check for understanding.
- "Coerced" change of physicians? Confront the issue directly; empathize with the patient.
- Dueling agendas? Confront the issue directly; explain the options and limits of care, while respecting the patient's experience and expectations.

These lead to better patient care and greater satisfaction, and they can be accomplished efficiently.

Other issues pertinent to primary care interviewing include concerns about preventive health care, confidentiality, truthfulness in the day-to-day practice of medicine, and malpractice suits.

- In preventive health care, the interview is important both diagnostically (establishing the patient's risk factors) and therapeutically (counseling for behavior change).
- Confidentiality is a primary value in medicine, but not an absolute one.
- Patient advocacy is an important part of primary care practice, but respect for patients and social institutions requires that advocacy be based on truthfulness.
- The most effective way to prevent malpractice suits is to enhance patient satisfaction. The best defensive medicine is good communication.

References

1. Levinson W, Stiles WB, Inui TS, Engle R. Physician frustration in communicating with patients. *Med Care* 1993; 31:285–295.
2. Beckman HB, Frankel RM. The effect of physician behavior on the collection of data. *Ann Intern Med* 1984; 101:692–696.
3. White J, Levinson W, Roter D. "Oh by the way . . .": The closing moments of the medical visit. *J Gen Intern Med* 1994; 9:24–28.
4. Hippocrates, translated by Jones WHS. The Loeb Classical Library, Cambridge MA, Harvard University Press, 1923.
5. Beckman HB, Markakis KM, Suchman AL, Frankel RM. The doctor-patient relationship and malpractice. *Arch Intern Med* 1994; 154:1365–1370.
6. Shapiro RS, Simpson DE, Lawrence SL, et al. A survey of sued and nonsued physicians and suing patients. *Arch Intern Med* 1989; 149:2190–2196.
7. Vincent C, Young M, Phillips A. Why do people sue doctors? A study of patients and relatives taking legal action. *Lancet* 1994; 343:1609–1613.

Suggested Readings

Bergh K. Time use and physicians' exploration of the reason for the office visit. *Fam Med* 1996; 28:264–270.

Bertakis KD, Roter D, Putnam SM. The relationship of physician medical interview style to patient satisfaction. *J Fam Pract* 1991; 32:175–181.

Emanuel EJ, Dubler NN. Preserving the physician-patient relationship in the era of managed care. *JAMA* 1995; 273:323–329.

Gordon GH, Baker L, Levinson W. Physician-patient communication in managed care. *West J Med* 1995; 163:527–531.

Inui TS. What are the sciences of relationship-centered primary care? *J Fam Pract* 1996; 42:171–177.

Leopold N, Cooper J, Clancy C. Sustained partnership in primary care. *J Fam Pract* 1996; 42:129–137.

CHAPTER 10

Seal Up the Mouth
of Outrage

• • •

INTERACTIVE PROBLEMS
IN INTERVIEWING

Seal up the mouth of outrage for a while

Till we can clear these ambiguities

And know their spring, their head, their true descent . . .

William Shakespeare,

Prince of Verona in *Romeo and Juliet*, Act V, Scene 3

In our interactive model of the medical interview, both the interviewer and patient play an active role in generating data that are as accurate and precise as possible. Sometimes even a novice finds it easy: the patient is alert, helpful, concise, and spontaneous; the problem is relatively straightforward; and there are no awkward elements such as a sexual problem. We want a story that is clear, internally consistent, logical, and not fictional. Sometimes, however, the interviewer—and usually the patient also—becomes aware that things are not going well. We label particular patients or situations as "difficult" when they present problems for us. The problems might arise from the patient, from the interviewer, from the topic under discussion, or from extraneous events. We have discussed earlier in this book that observer bias and instrument precision play a part in any medical observation, whether a gallium scan, auscultation of the heart, or generation of a medical history. There are ways of improving the quality of each of these observations even

TABLE 10–1 DIFFICULT PATIENT-DOCTOR INTERACTIONS

1. Process problems
  a. Technical impairments (Chap. 2)
    (1) Organic (delirium or dementia)
    (2) Language barrier
  b. Style impairments (Chap. 3)
    (1) Reticence
    (2) Rambling
    (3) Vagueness
2. Topical problems (Chaps. 5 and 6)
  a. Drugs, alcohol, diet, and smoking
  b. Sexual functioning
  c. Positive review of systems
3. Interactive styles
  a. Dependent, demanding
  b. Orderly, controlled
  c. Dramatic
  d. Long-suffering, masochistic
  e. Guarded, paranoid
  f. Superior
	4. Somatization
	5. Difficult feelings
	  a. The patient's feelings
	    (1) Anxiety
	    (2) Anger
	    (3) Depression
	    (4) Denial
	  b. Patients' and interviewers' feelings
	    about each other

SOURCE: Adapted from Kahana and Bibring.[1]

in the presence of adverse circumstances; for example, the examiner can close the window or jiggle the earpieces of the stethoscope to improve perception of a murmur. The same is true with the difficult patient situation; remedial actions improve the outcome.

Table 10–1 presents a taxonomy of difficult doctor-patient interactions, including a number of process and topical problems that have been presented in earlier chapters as challenges that regularly arise during the course of routine medical interactions. Sociocultural issues fit more appropriately into our discussion of health beliefs (see Chap. 14) and negotiation (see Chap. 15). In this chapter we discuss patients' interactive styles, somatization, and difficult feelings. These divisions are arbitrary for the sake of clarification and discussion; remember that we rarely see them in pure form and that clinicians also have styles and feelings (or sometimes just a bad day) that interact to produce difficult interviews.

INTERACTIVE STYLES

Occasionally the patient's interactive or personality style interferes with obtaining objective and precise data. Of course, everyone has a personality style, but under stress, such as that which accompanies illness, distinct coping behaviors may become exaggerated or even dysfunctional. Identifying a particular style gives you important information about how patients perceive their illness, how they "filter" historic data, and how they generally interact with other people. Kahana and Bibring, in a classic paper,[1] presented observations on personality styles and suggested ways of coping with them during the interview in order to maximize your ability to obtain accurate data. The styles are:

- Dependent and demanding
- Orderly and controlled
- Dramatizing or manipulative
- Long-suffering or masochistic
- Guarded or paranoid
- Superior

This is a useful classification to orient our discussion, although we rarely see people who exhibit a truly "pure" style.

The Dependent, Demanding Style

This person strives to impress the clinician with the urgent quality of all of his or her requests. The patient needs special attention, great reassurance, and constant advice. You may first see an optimistic, compliant, and "good" patient but soon find that the patient expects a limitless amount of attention and care. Groves[2] described this type of person as one of his "hateful patients" and used the term "dependent clinger." When the patient's need for "boundless interest and abundant care" is unmet, he or she may become depressed or withdrawn or may blame the clinician in a complaining or vengeful way. Trying to meet every demand may lead to exhaustion.

In many acutely ill patients, dependent tendencies temporarily come to the fore and should be met with active, empathic, and generous care directed toward the patient's physical and emotional comfort. When this pattern becomes exaggerated or chronic, however, you must set limits, such as by stating specific follow-up appointments, supplying specific written instructions, and insisting that the patient clearly understand his or her responsibility. It is important for the beginning clinician to learn to "protect the patient from promises that cannot be kept and from illusions that are bound to shatter."[2] This is not the patient for whom you should arrange special appointment times, permit repeated phone calls after hours for nonemergency problems, or make repeated calls to the pharmacy for prescriptions that all seem to run out on different days.

Similarly, within the interview itself, the goal is to set limits for the patient so that the basic task at hand, obtaining accurate data, can be accomplished. This means that the patient must understand the limits of the "contract" (e.g., you are a student, albeit an interested one, doing a medical history), as well as the need to discuss specific types of information in order for you to understand the patient's problems. Useful techniques include the following:

- Suspect this problem in new patients who make you feel that you are the only one who has ever cared about them or understood their illness.

- Avoid making promises that you cannot keep, such as solving a nursing or insurance problem.

- Give the patient responsibility with a statement such as "Perhaps you can talk with the nurses about your pain medication."

- Remind the patient that your time is limited, despite the fact that you are interested in his or her story. Try a statement such as "You certainly have a lot of important problems, but since my time is so short, I'd like to get back to the reason you came into the hospital."

- Do not take credit for remission in the patient's symptoms, as you will likely be blamed for a relapse, which is sure to follow. Give responsibility to the patient with a statement such as "You're the one who did what was necessary to get better."

The Orderly and Controlled Style

Some patients, when under stress, cope by gaining as much knowledge as possible about their situation, not only to deal with their problem rationally but also to handle their anxiety. They are punctual for appointments, conscientious in taking medications, and preoccupied with the right way and the wrong way of carrying out your instructions. Sickness threatens these patients with loss of control. They may present with a list of carefully thought-out questions or a precise diary of their symptoms. They find the scientific medical approach congenial to their way of thinking and respond well to the professional, systematic sequence of history taking, physical diagnosis, laboratory studies, and therapy.

Because patients of this type are often on the same "wavelength" as the health professional, they do not appear to present a difficult situation. However, you must be careful to explain their problems thoroughly and describe carefully any laboratory tests or procedures. Also, if you pause a little longer over auscultation of the heart or inquire into an area of history seemingly unrelated to their problem, they may suffer excessive anxiety unless you take care to explain why you are doing these things. These patients must be permitted to take charge of their own medical care and be given positive feedback about their efforts and abilities.

Within the interview, this type of patient finds it helpful if the interviewer has an orderly and systematic approach, with frequent explanations as to what is happening. Summarizing what you have heard reassures this patient that you are listening and that you are not missing any of the details the patient considers vital to making the diagnosis. This patient will be re-assured by note taking (he or she does not want you to forget anything important) but will be alarmed if you suddenly write something down when you have not been writing all along. If you are asked why you are pursuing a particular line of questioning, make it clear that the purpose is routine or that you want to clarify an item; do not alarm this type of patient by re-vealing all the vague diagnostic hypotheses running around in your head that led to a particular question. Here is an example:

Dr: How have you been?

Pt: I was trying to remember if I was supposed to call you. I think, I don't remember when I called last and now I couldn't remember if I was supposed to call you again or not.

Dr: Well, that's fine. I just was hoping that you hadn't tried and not gotten through or something like that. I understand you got new glasses. Has that helped?

Pt: I don't see the slightest difference.

Dr: You're not happy because you're having trouble seeing?

Pt: I'm not happy because I don't see as well as I would like to see. I can't see numbers well.

Dr: Does the eye doctor give you an explanation?

Pt: Well, he keeps talking. He talks to me, referring, speaking to me as "your cataract" and I said to him plainly, I said, "You referred to my cataract many times. You have never told me I have a cataract. Do I?" And he said everyone over 30 years old has a cataract. So that's . . .

Dr: So that's really not an answer. So you don't know whether it's the cataract, whether you have it in both eyes, or whether there's some other problem.

Pt: I don't know and I can't get a straight answer.

And later in the interview,

Pt: I wanted to tell you about that and I'm trying to think if there is anything else I should tell you. I don't remember anything. Of course, some of the problems are getting worse but I don't consider that something that wasn't expected. I assume that's what we should expect. Everything else is pretty much under control.

Notice how carefully this patient uses her words. When the physician says, "You're having trouble seeing?" she "corrects" this wording with "I don't see as well as I would like to see." She does not say, "There isn't anything else I should tell you"; she says instead, "I don't remember anything" (and this is interesting, because she is elderly and knows she has a little trouble with her recent memory). Notice her concern with doing the right thing, being compliant ("I was trying to remember if I was supposed to call you"). Consider the importance to her of explanations and how disquieted she is by the ophthalmologist's evasiveness ("I can't get a straight answer"). Despite the fact that "some of the problems are getting worse," she tolerates that because "I don't consider that something that wasn't expected." What is good is that "everything else is pretty much under control." Note how the physician is able to clarify her concerns while avoiding explanations about a problem with which he is unfamiliar (i.e., her eye problem, for which she sees someone else).

The Dramatic Style

This type of patient may first present as interesting and charming, even when he or she dramatizes and makes global statements about symptoms: The pain is "the worst pain I have ever had . . . it's with me all the time, day and night, nothing seems to help. . . . I haven't been able to sleep in weeks. . . ." This person may have a great need to be at stage center and may resent the doctor's interest in other duties and other patients. "To the dramatizing emotionally involved kind of person, sickness may feel like a personal defect; it means being weak and unattractive, unappreciated, and unsuccessful."[1] These patients are frequently characterized as dramatic and manipulative and sometimes, particularly when dealing with a clinician of the opposite sex, as seductive.

We have emphasized the importance of allowing the patient to tell the story in his or her own words, with some direction from the interviewer but without the high-control style that produces poor data. There are times, however, when the issue of control is central to the interview process; the patient wants too much control, and you are unable to obtain the information you need. Sometimes the problem permeates the entire history; at other times, the problem is limited to a particular part of the history. For instance, a patient with a drug problem may steer the discussion into other areas every time you approach the question of substance abuse.

Sometimes the patient wants to control you and engages in a type of behavior not usually appropriate to a professional relationship, such as noticing your new watch or hairstyle, complimenting you on your good taste, or asking personal questions about your social relationships or sexual preference. Here are some guidelines for dealing with this type of behavior in the interview:

- Listen to and observe the patient as he or she demonstrates this type of behavior. Think: What does the patient wish to gain by this behavior?

- Control the urge to engage in open warfare for control of the interview by feeding back what you hear and clarifying points.

- Remain calm, gentle, and firm, using frequent summaries to regain or stay in control.

- Remain descriptive, not judgmental or evaluative; focus on the how, not the why. For example, "I've noticed that when I try to ask you about drug use you tend to change the subject," not "Why don't you answer my question?"

- Identify the strengths of the patient and feed them back by establishing a profile of the premorbid person, as well as of the patient you are currently interviewing.

- If the patient asks you a personal question or one you are uncomfortable about answering, try reflecting back to the patient with a statement such as "Well, we're really not here to talk about my opinion . . . I'm interested in hearing more about you. How did you handle that?"

- Reframe seductive behavior positively as one of the patient's many possible moves toward attaining goals in his or her life. For example, you can say, "I see that you enjoy being an attractive woman and you enjoy being with a man and being noticed by him and taken care of by him. How do you meet those needs in your life?" or "So you are a widower, how has that been for you?"

Taking a thorough history in a respectful atmosphere where you demonstrate you are in charge is the best way to build a solid relationship with the patient and to establish a treatment plan that will be acceptable.

The Long-Suffering, Masochistic Style

Groves[2] describes these patients as "help rejectors." They give a history of continual suffering from disease, disappointment, and other adversity. They see their lives as a sequence of bad luck. Often they disregard their own needs in order to do things for other people. Despite apparent humility, these patients may have a tendency to be exhibitionistic about their long-suffering fate. With regard to medical care, they feel that no treatment will help; when one symptom goes away, another appears in its place.

Simple reassurance and optimism will not be "bought" by the masochistic patient. Within the interview, avoid trying to talk the patient out of the severe nature of his or her suffering. Similarly, avoid overly optimistic or patronizing remarks such as "I'm sure you'll be feeling better in no time." Although this patient may not regard talking to a student or resident as therapeutic, he or she may like the idea of helping you by permitting you to do a history and physical. Accept the patient's pessimism with a statement such as "It sounds as though you don't think there is much hope of getting better."

Consider the following interchange with an 82-year-old woman who is experiencing failing abilities and is trying to care single-handedly for her severely demented 89-year-old spouse:

Dr: How have things been going for you?

Pt: Well, not much different. Same as usual. Same problems, same lack of solutions. I'm not saying that anyone would give me a different answer, but I still don't have to like it.

Dr: Yeah, you feel that you've gotten that answer to a lot of problems.

Pt: I feel that I've gotten that answer everywhere. Everything that I have problems with. Everything, that is, except Dr. Jackson, who wants to operate on my throat . . .

Dr: Which you don't want.

Pt: No. Pretty hopeless, isn't it.

Dr: Well, I think you're doing about as well as anyone could do.

Pt: Well, I don't know, maybe I am. Again I say it's not good enough, but I don't suppose there's any 'good enough' in a situation like that.

Dr: How do you feel about the medication right now? Do you think it's helped your spirits at all?

Pt: I like to believe it does. I can't be real sure because I don't know how I'd be feeling without it, but I try to imagine it soothes me some.

Dr: Good.

Pt: I don't think it's doing me any harm.

Dr: Good. What about getting some extra help at home? Have you made any progress with that?

Pt: I don't know. The reason I have resisted is because I had a sister-in-law who could not live alone and she had an endless succession of people that I know stole from her and robbed her.

Dr: The best thing is to get either someone that you know well or a person who is recommended by someone you trust.

Pt: That's true, but I don't think that person exists.

Dr: I wish there were something I could do to help.

Pt: I don't expect you to have solutions. It's just how things are. Nothing can change.

This kind of interchange is enough to make any physician feel pretty hopeless as well. Note the patient's repeated return to the theme of no solutions. The most optimistic she gets (and it is not much) is "I like to believe" that the antidepressant she has been taking is helpful, at least "I don't think it's doing me any harm." The physician finally gives up making suggestions and begins to share the patient's pessimism: "I wish there were something I could do to help." The patient, in turn, paradoxically reassures the physician ("I don't expect you to have solutions").

The Guarded, Paranoid Style

Some patients are inclined to be suspicious of health-care professionals and the medical care establishment. They may present a long list of slights from others and openly point out how the illness was mishandled; or they will blame others for their illness. During stress, the patient may become "even more fearful, guarded, suspicious, quarrelsome and controlling of others."[1] The clinician may find himself or herself always feeling "on guard" during the interview, as if to avoid being "caught" in a competitive relationship.

It is important to give this patient clear explanations of your strategy for diagnosis and treatment. If you are a student or house officer, pay particular attention to identifying your role and clarifying its limitations. These patients may make provocative statements, but arguing with them or ignoring their suspicious attitudes does not help. The best approach is to maintain a friendly and courteous attitude while acknowledging the patient's beliefs, even though you do not necessarily agree with them.

Within the interview, a frequent problem with these patients is their stated disgust with those caring for them—namely, physicians and nurses—and you are guilty by association. The patient may say with great exasperation, "All I want to know is if I've had a heart attack . . . Why doesn't my doctor tell me yes or no?" It is rarely useful to try to unravel such a question, in part because the answers may not be there and in part because the patient may think that you are taking sides either with or against him or her. It is better to acknowledge and accept the patient's suspicions with a statement such as "It must be terribly frustrating, not knowing." Then try to proceed with the history by reminding the patient that while there is nothing you can do to help with that particular problem, "I am interested in hearing more about the symptoms that brought you to the hospital."

The Superior Style

These patients have strong self-confidence and may appear smug, vain, or even grandiose. Their behavior in the medical care situation is often that identified by Groves[2] as the "entitled demander." They may demand the most senior physician or the most well-known subspecialist, and may be very condescending or arrogant toward house officers, students, and their primary care physicians. They may attempt to control the physician, not only by making many demands but also sometimes by threatening litigation. As Groves[2] writes, "Entitlement serves for some persons the functions that faith and hope serve in better adjusted ones." Often, this patient may react to situations that occur in the hospital with anger and hostility—anger that can impinge upon you as caregiver. The suggestions presented later in this chapter for dealing with anger are also appropriate for this patient.

Although for some patients this style is pervasive, more often a patient suddenly makes demands on the health-care professional that he or she would not ordinarily make. Consider this example of a young actor who had never had any difficult interactions with his physician until he developed a "cold or flu or something which normally I would just wait until it went away except I'm involved in a show right now." The dialogue continues:

Pt: And it's the leading role in a rather important production and we open this Thursday (clears throat) and I went into this cold.

Dr: You open this coming Thursday.

Pt: And I went into a cold; it feels like it's been in my system for about 2 weeks, but then on about Thursday it started clearing up. Then because of an audition Friday morning I got like 6 hours of sleep. Friday I started to feel coldish, Saturday I felt terrible, yesterday I felt terrible, so I feel I just need some kind of prescription . . . to be able to deal with it.

So this patient who would "normally just wait" suddenly feels entitled to treatment for a problem that is self-limited and that has no definitive therapy. It is as though the patient is saying, "I know there is no cure for a cold, but since I'm the lead in an important production you must make an exception and cure me." This sounds paradoxical and illogical. In such a situation, the physician might respond:

Dr: There's no cure for the common cold! Actors are no different from anyone else!

Pt: If you won't help me I'll find someone who will.

But things go better if the doctor says:

Dr: I can understand your concern, what with this production and all. As you know, there's no cure for the common cold. But why don't I take a look at you and maybe I can recommend something to get the symptoms under control so you'll feel in better form.

Pt: Okay. I sure hope there's something you can do.

SOMATIZATION

The Nature of Somatization

You will encounter certain patients whose symptoms are legion but in whom no "organic" etiology for these symptoms can be identified. Some of these patients have relatively brief somatic problems that resolve over time. Some have recurrent and multiple physical complaints that span many years, many doctors, and many diagnostic work-ups, yet you cannot make any pathophysiologic sense out of the story as a whole. Sometimes the patient will tell you that "Doctors have never been able to find anything" and that "they said it was all in my head." Other patients in this group will have been provided with a series of diagnoses and treatments: gallbladder disease followed by cholecystectomy for abdominal pain, uterine fibroids followed by hysterectomy for pelvic pain, degenerative disc disease followed by laminectomy for back pain, or abdominal adhesions (from previous surgery) followed by yet another operation for lysis of adhesions (for the now-recurrent abdominal pain). Despite diagnosed disorders to which to ascribe symptoms, patients improve only partially and temporarily when treated and soon develop new symptoms. Such patients suffer real pain and often develop real disability, even though their problems appear to resist the ordinary disease categories.

These patients are "somatizers." Somatization is a process whereby people experience and express emotional discomfort or psychosocial stress in the language of physical symptoms. As Nathaniel Hawthorne wrote, "A bodily disease, which we look upon as whole and entire within itself, may, after all, be but a symptom of some ailment in the spiritual part."

This process may occur in the absence of other disorders (primary somatization), or it may be associated with other medical or psychiatric conditions (secondary somatization). We consider somatization here for three reasons:

- Patients with functional somatic symptoms are frequently encountered in practice, and they often consume large amounts of interview time.

- Somatizing patients are difficult to interview.

- The medical interview and thorough review of the past medical history are critical to the diagnosis of somatoform disorders.

Table 10–2 presents a differential diagnosis of somatization as a psychiatric disorder. In the somatoform disorders (hypochondriasis, conversion, psychogenic pain, somatization, and undifferentiated somatoform disorder), the process of somatization is a primary feature, and specific diagnostic criteria apply. A larger group of patients suffer functional somatic symptoms but do not meet *Diagnostic and Statistical Manual of Mental Disorders,* ed. 4

TABLE 10-2   DIFFERENTIAL DIAGNOSIS OF SOMATIZATION

1. Occult physical disease
   a. Syndromes of unknown etiology
      (1) Fibromyalgia or fibromyositis
      (2) Chronic fatigue syndrome
      (3) Mitral valve prolapse syndrome
   b. Diseases with subtle, multisystem
      manifestations (e.g., systemic lupus
      erythematosus, multiple sclerosis,
      hyperparathyroidism)
2. Secondary somatization
   a. Secondary to known chronic disease
   b. Secondary to other psychiatric
      disorders
      (1) Major depression
      (2) Adjustment reactions
      (3) Alcohol or other substance
          abuse
      (4) Panic and other anxiety
          disorders
3. Primary somatization
   a. Transient functional somatic
      symptoms
   b. Somatoform disorders
      (1) Somatization disorder
      (2) Hypochondriasis
      (3) Conversion reaction
      (4) Psychogenic pain disorder
      (5) Undifferentiated somatoform
          disorder
4. Factitious disease

(*DSM-IV*) criteria for one of these conditions or for any other psychiatric disorder. These patients may be said to have an amplifying somatic style. Table 10-3 presents a more general survey of the manifestations of somatization in clinical practice. Somatizers use more medical services, require more sick leave and disability, and perceive themselves as less healthy than medically ill patients. Their interpersonal relationships, families, and ways of looking at the world are all affected by unending sickliness. Medical care itself provides a positive feedback loop that validates the patient's sickliness, creating new anxiety ("After all, if no one can find out what it is, it must be something strange and terrible"), and causes additional suffering.

TABLE 10-3   MANIFESTATIONS OF SOMATIZATION IN CLINICAL PRACTICE

1. Selective focus on somatic symptoms of a psychiatric disorder (e.g., the fatigue of depression or palpitations of panic)
2. Amplification of somatic symptoms of organic illness
3. Use of somatic symptoms in the absence of demonstrable organic disease to avoid dysphoric affect or intrapsychic conflict, or to manipulate social environment for personal "gain"
4. Selective focus on psychophysiologic symptoms with denial or minimization of life problems that precipitate or exacerbate the symptoms
5. Expression of somatic complaints as a culturally sanctioned idiom of distress

SOURCE: Adapted from Katon et al.[3]

The following pages briefly consider (1) the diagnosis of somatization in the medical history and (2) somatization as it relates to the doctor-patient interaction.

Somatization in the Medical History

We distinguish among three types of "symptom generation," all of which may be considered manifestations of somatization:

- **Patients may amplify symptoms** of acute or chronic organic disease, or may preferentially report somatic symptoms (while de-emphasizing emotional symptoms) of psychiatric conditions. The latter process results in, for example, "masked" depression, a condition often poorly diagnosed and treated.[4] Patients with masked depression may visit their doctors with a chief complaint of fatigue and be almost unaware of their low mood. In such cases, the interview must be directed toward identifying those "unamplified" or suppressed symptoms that complete the diagnostic pattern. In fact, primary care patients who suffer from major depression usually do report their affective symptoms if asked directly.[5]

- **Patients may report psychophysiologic disturbances** (e.g., headaches, tachycardia, palpitations, or irregular bowel movements) mediated through autonomic or other known pathophysiologic mechanisms. Many patients have these sorts of problems, and each can be diagnosed as a separate syndrome. Examples include irritable bowel syndrome, fibromyalgia, and premenstrual syndrome. However, if you obtain a history of multiple, recurrent, or disabling psychophysiologic syndromes, give some attention to the process of somatization. It is important not to lose sight of the forest because you are carefully studying every tree.

- **Patients may experience actual conversion symptoms.** These symptoms serve a symbolic function in the patient's life (i.e., they actually represent or replace an emotion), rather than being nonspecific responses to conflict or life's stress. Consequently, conversion symptoms do not necessarily correspond to known physiologic mechanisms or anatomic distributions. These symptoms often develop acutely (an important historical feature) and simply do not make sense to the doctor. The patient's description of a severe deficit (e.g., complete loss of feeling in the left leg and paralysis of the right arm) does not correspond at all with the physical signs or what is anatomically possible. Because these symptoms originate in the unconscious, their symbolic meaning is hidden from the patient.

Persons with recurrent or persistent somatization may experience all three of these types of symptoms. Most often, however, you will find amplified or

TABLE 10–4 CHARACTERISTICS OF PATIENTS AND SYMPTOMS SUGGESTIVE OF SOMATIZATION

1. The symptom's description is vague, inconsistent, or bizarre.
2. The symptoms persist despite apparently adequate medical therapy.
3. The illness begins in the context of a psychologically meaningful setting (e.g., death of relative, conflict with spouse, or job promotion).
4. The patient denies any emotional distress or psychological role of the symptoms.
5. The patient has engaged in polydoctoring and/or has had polysurgery.
6. There is evidence of an associated psychiatric disorder.
7. The patient has features suggesting a hysterical personality style.
8. Discussion reveals that the patient attributes an idiosyncratic meaning to his or her symptoms.
9. The patient has difficulty describing emotions or inner processes in words.

SOURCE: Adapted and abridged from Lipkin.[6]

psychophysiologic complaints, either separately or in combination. True conversion symptoms, although not rare, are infrequent. Virtually any specific symptom can be a manifestation of somatization; it need not be a weird, complex, or inexplicable complaint. In fact, when evaluating a patient for somatization, you should concentrate on the pattern, logic, and context of the symptom, rather than trying to decide whether dizziness, for example, is more likely than dysuria to represent somatization. You should look for "positive" features in the medical history that suggest somatization, rather than simply taking the "negative" approach of ruling out every conceivable organic disease. Table 10–4 presents nine such positive characteristics. If two or three of these are present, you should consider the hypothesis that the patient's symptoms are at least partly attributable to somatization. You can test this hypothesis by directing your interview toward establishing whether additional features are present. For example, given a vague symptom that persists despite therapy, you might be particularly careful to explore the symptom's cognitive or emotional meaning ("What do you think is causing this?") and to search for evidence of psychiatric disorders such as major depression.

Somatization in the Doctor-Patient Interaction

What can you do within the interview for the somatizing patient? Consistent application of good listening and responding skills is the basis of any effective interview, laying the groundwork for effective therapy. Although difficult, it is necessary to build a trusting relationship, to validate his or her suffering as a medical problem, to provide a clear explanation of symptoms, and to engage active patient participation in the treatment. The following

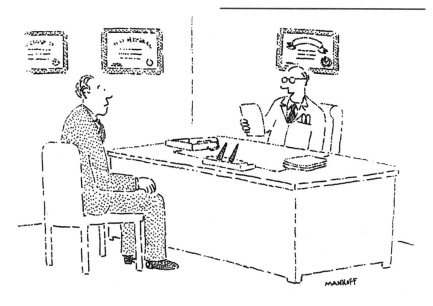

*"Well, this is a very impressive résumé, young man. I think
you're going to make a fine patient."*

Drawing by Mankoff; © 1988
The New Yorker Magazine, Inc.
Used by permission.

are a few specific pointers useful in early encounters with somatizing patients:

- In the initial assessment, obtain a complete patient profile, including functional status and family interactions, even though the patient wants only to discuss his or her symptoms.

- Likewise, pay particular attention to details of the past medical history (see above cartoon). This may require obtaining the names and addresses of numerous doctors and sending for the patient's records. Somatizers often fragment their health care. Because she doesn't think it is relevant, a patient may not volunteer the names of her cardiologist and her dermatologist when she is seeing you for a gastrointestinal complaint. One of the authors saw a patient with somatization disorder who at one time had regular, ongoing relationships with 12 doctors: two gastroenterologists, two pain control specialists, a neurosurgeon, an otolaryngologist, a cardiologist, a urologist, a general surgeon, a family doctor, a general internist, and a psychiatrist.

- Establish goals with the patient. In particular, if there are multiple symptoms expressed in the interview, agree on which one(s) need attention first. If a symptom is chronic, point out that a similarly long period of treatment may be required before the symptom improves or resolves. Sometimes a "contract" is helpful: you agree to address the patient's concerns, and the patient agrees to be reassured if there is no cause for alarm.

- Avoid "vague references" (see p. 168). Even though you may not be sure of a symptom's underlying etiology, you can still explain in physiologic terms both its operation and your plan for treatment.

- Speak of the body, not of the mind. Many patients will have been told by doctors, "It's all in your head." It is generally not useful to explain the symptom as something that originates in the mind because this approach makes the patient feel that the symptom is not "real." When talking about "stress" or "tension," relate it to the autonomic nervous system, which, in turn, causes the disagreeable sensation or symptom.

- In each encounter, focus some attention on healthy talk (e.g., the patient's strengths and activities), rather than concentrating only on symptoms. This will be difficult at first because the patient may find any talk other than symptom talk irrelevant and perhaps suspicious. Genuine empathic concern often can break through and allow the somatizer to be more open with you.

- Examine the patient. There are two reasons to repeat selective, but careful, physical examinations. First, you do not want to miss signs of organic disease that may develop at any time in anyone's body, including that of a somatizer. Second, because somatizers are focused on their bodies, your attention to the body is evidence that you take their concerns seriously. It helps validate their symptoms and thus helps you develop a healing relationship.

In general, good care for the somatizing patient requires a management strategy that includes:

- Explicit rules and guidelines
- Regularly scheduled office visits
- Careful monitoring of health status
- Supportive discussion or counseling, education, and appropriate symptomatic medication
- Consultation with a psychiatrist or psychologist when appropriate

DIFFICULT FEELINGS IN THE MEDICAL INTERVIEW

Sometimes the patient's feelings or emotions produce behaviors that interfere with transmitting adequate information of the kind you need for a precise and accurate history: an angry patient may not wish to speak with you at all, a depressed patient may say too little, and a denying patient may be unable to reveal the very symptoms that are so terrifying to him. Such situations often have us feeling several things at once: we may be frustrated at the difficulty in obtaining the history, yet feel sorry for the depressed patient;

be concerned about maintaining a professional attitude, yet feel defensive or outraged at the angry patient; or feel pleased at the gratitude shown by the seductive patient, yet upset at being manipulated. When we sense strong emotions occurring in the interview, we often try to ignore them with the excuse that it is really not our job as a clinician to deal with the patient's emotions.

Although it may not be your job to treat the cancer patient's depression or the multiple sclerosis patient's denial, it is your job to do a good medical interview. When such feelings get in the way, they need to be acknowledged so that the interview can proceed efficiently and accurately. Experienced clinicians find that empathic responses not only help the patient feel understood but also facilitate the interview, from the point of view of both time (it takes less time) and accuracy (the patient gives better data).

General Strategies for Dealing with Difficult Feelings

When feelings interfere with obtaining the history, be sure to observe carefully the basics of any good interview:

- If you are a student, make sure you have the patient's permission to do the interview and that he or she understands the contract with you:
    - Empathize with the patient's position: "I know many doctors have already come in and bothered you. . . ."
    - Elicit the patient's permission, perhaps with a question such as "Is it all right?" If the answer is yes, show your appreciation. If the answer is no, accept the patient's noncooperation and ask for the reasons in a noncombative way, recognizing the patient's right to refuse.
    - Inform the patient gently of your obligation to do the interview, without attempting to convince or control him or her. Give control to the patient by indicating your willingness to compromise within your limits, such as by asking, "Would it help if I came back in an hour? If I rearranged your pillows? If I talked softer (louder), faster (slower)? If I stood (sat)?"
- Listen, giving the patient time to respond, particularly when the subject under discussion is hard for the patient to talk about:
    - Ask open-ended questions and observe the total communication, including words, gestures, facial expressions, and voice quality.
    - Wait for the patient to finish his or her thought or sentence, even if he or she hesitates or stumbles over words.
- Summarize periodically both the symptom content and the feeling content. Specific uses of summaries include:
    - To regain control if the patient has wandered off the topic or you are feeling confused. For example, "You are telling me a lot

about yourself. Let me tell you what I understand so far, because I will want to ask you a specific question."

- To prepare the way for a potentially threatening question. For example, "You have had a lot of back pain, and from what you tell me, it has also made you quite depressed. . . . Has it affected your marriage? Your sex life?"
- To clarify and remain "in sync" with the patient, particularly when you notice that the patient feels upset or misunderstood. For example, "Just now, as you were describing your pain, you got a very worried look on your face. . . . Did I say something that upset you?"

- Use the interchangeable empathic response to show that you understand exactly. Try to describe precisely in your own words the patient's symptoms as well as the intensity of emotions being expressed. Look to the patient for confirmation of your statement and acknowledge any corrections. For example:

Dr: So as I understand it, you've been having this pain in your chest for the past 2 to 3 months, and you notice it when you go jogging, and you're a little worried about what's causing it? (Doctor looks up at patient.)

Pt: Well, it's not pain exactly, more a discomfort. And actually I'm more than a little worried. My father dropped dead of a heart attack when he was 43, and I'm 42.

Dr: I see. So you're worried that the same thing might happen to you?

Pt: Yeah, I'd really like you to take a cardiogram on me, doc.

- If you feel lost, acknowledge it as a fact, not as a criticism of the patient. Then proceed to ask the patient to help you: "I'm confused about this, can you help me?" or "I did not quite understand this point, would you help me?"

We will next consider patient anxiety, anger, depression, and denial and, in each case, suggest specific approaches to supplement those we have already discussed.

Anxiety

Every illness produces at least some anxiety, if not outright fear, in the patient. Common sources of anxiety are feelings of helplessness, fear of pain and disability, inability to accept warmth or tenderness, fear of expressing anger, and, of course, uncertainty about the future. When people become anxious, they tend to intensify their customary ways of coping with the world: a compulsive patient may become more particular, and a paranoid patient may become more guarded. Signs of anxiety that you may observe in the interview include facial flushing, sweating, rapid speech, cold hands, fidgeting, or even trembling. The anxious patient may be difficult to interview until the anxiety has been discussed.

All patients are anxious and, to some extent, fearful about a medical interview. Some ways you can help the anxious patient are:

- Be unhurried and calm in your manner.

- Sympathize, but remember that too much sympathy may magnify the patient's fears.

- Be very specific as to what you expect of the patient: what clothing the patient should remove or what position the patient should assume and where.

- Tell the patient that some anxiety is normal and appropriate: most patients feel this way and it is okay.

- Some patients express their anxiety by asking what you think is causing their symptoms. When this happens, it is appropriate to remind the patient that you are a student or that you have not completed your evaluation. In addition, you can explore the patient's concerns by asking "Have you asked your doctor? (And if not, why not?)" or "What do you think is going on?"

Consider this case example. A 57-year-old woman saw her family physician for an annual examination. Doctors made her nervous and the thought of a visit, even on this day when she had no particularly worrisome symptoms, made her nervous. Her red lipstick was coated with antacid as she entered the office; she was so distraught that her stomach felt queasy. It was clear (in retrospect) that just showing up for the examination was a major effort for her. Everything, fortunately, was in order. The physician had only one prescription for her:

Dr: Everything is fine. I have only one recommendation, and that is that I'd like you to get a mammogram.

Pt: Oh my God! You mean I've got cancer? Not my breast!

Dr: No, no, of course not. No, I recommend a mammogram for all my patients over the age of 50. It's routine.

And, as though the physician were not leveling with her:

Pt: I couldn't stand to lose a breast; chemotherapy is awful. I already have thinning hair, you know; chemotherapy makes that worse. No, won't do that—I can't.

In retrospect, this patient's fragile adaptation to her encounter with a physician was shattered by one suggestion of a routine screening test. She seemed to believe that the recommendation was particular, not routine, despite her doctor's protests to the contrary. If we look back at how the clinician introduced the idea, we notice what may have seemed to the patient to be a contradiction: "Everything is fine . . . get a mammogram." For this anxiety-ridden patient, "If 'everything is fine,' why do I need a mammogram?" The physician might have been able to achieve the aim of getting her to have a mammogram (which, by the way, she never agreed to) by saying:

- Dr: Everything's fine. Your exam is completely normal. Just like you come for a Pap test because you know that's routine in all women, so we routinely recommend a mammogram for all women your age, and you mentioned that you had not had one done for a while.

In this instance, the physician is more reassuring because she is specific about what is "fine" ("Your exam is completely normal"), frames the routine nature of the mammogram in a concrete way to which the patient can relate (i.e., by comparing it to the routine Pap test), and anticipates the patient's worry by explaining the reason for the test before the patient can spin a fantasy of calamity.

Anger

Although a patient's anxiety may lead us to feel sympathetic toward him or her, we usually find anger more difficult to handle. Patients behave in a hostile manner for many different reasons. Most of the time the reasons have nothing to do with us personally; rather, they relate to the patient's own situation, such as inconsiderate care by hospital staff, failure to communicate, or the patient's unique response to his or her illness, disability, or prognosis. What makes one patient depressed may make another patient angry, and the seemingly angry patient may, in reality, be depressed. Some ways to handle anger include:

- Recognize and acknowledge anger with a statement such as "I can see (hear or feel) you are angry and frustrated," or "Waiting so long makes most people angry." If you are not sure that what you are hearing is anger, ask, "Are you feeling angry?" Try not to "accuse" the patient of being angry.

- Accept the anger by continuing to listen to the patient while explaining the situation in a neutral fashion, even though a logical explanation will not necessarily change the patient's feelings. Do not take sides.

- Explore the contributing factors and identify the underlying feelings, such as fear, hurt, disappointment, or powerlessness. Accept the patient's reason even if you do not personally agree with it. Remember, there is always a reason, although it may not be immediately evident.

- If the patient's anger is justifiably directed at you, acknowledge your mistake. We are always learning; mistakes are unavoidable; we learn from our mistakes and correct them. If the patient's anger is not directed at you, help the patient recognize ways he or she can deal with the anger-provoking situations. For example:

Pt: You're just as insensitive as the rest of 'em.

Dr: I guess that was a foolish question to ask. Now that I understand you a little better, do you think we could start over?

Another patient was angry after being interviewed in front of a group of residents at a psychiatric case conference. She is talking to her physician following the conference:

Pt: I now know what it's like to be poor. I never would have been at that conference if I had my own private doctor. I know what it's like to be a guinea pig. That doctor asked about my early childhood when what I needed was someone to find out what's been going on over the last 10 years and how tough life has been for me so that he could help me. I thought he would be able to give me something to help my nerves right now, not just talk about my grandmother.

Although this patient reminds us of the entitled demander (see p. 191), and indeed may be one, she is clear, if we listen, about what is upsetting her. She is focused on how she feels at present and is looking for relief from feelings that are unpleasant. Talking about what seemed to her to be ancient history confused and frustrated her. The conference ended apparently without a prescription or clear plan of action, and although the physician was trying to remedy the situation, the patient may not have known that. Here an explanation and an acknowledgment of her feelings are in order:

Dr: It certainly must seem strange to talk about old things when you feel so bad now and want relief. I can certainly understand your frustration. Actually, the reason I wanted to talk with you is to discuss what to do next to get you to feel better. Because Dr. Smith had some good ideas that I think we should try. In fact, he suggested some medication that he thinks will be helpful, and I think so, too.

The other aspect of her anger was a sense of being on display or of being experimented with (perhaps two sides of the same coin). She may have been surprised by the conference format, requiring her to sit in front of a room full of strange doctors she had never met before. Someone should have prepared her for what was to occur; if no one did, her physician can only apologize:

Dr: I'm sorry, I guess I didn't really explain very well what was supposed to happen to you. I'm sorry you felt uncomfortable. But I did learn a lot about you which I think will help me to take better care of you.
Pt: Okay. What I really need is to feel better.

Depression

Depression may be a manifestation of a diagnosable psychiatric disorder, a response to recent tragedy (such as death of a spouse), an expression of a generally pessimistic approach to life, or a transient feeling state. Major depressive disorder may be the underlying problem in a substantial percentage of those patients who complain to their physicians of fatigue, weakness, lack of energy, insomnia, backache, or headache, but depression as a response to illness is also common. Depressive characteristics include feelings of worthlessness, hopelessness, apathy, and guilt, together with a profoundly empty and lonely feeling. These are manifest in the patient's manner, tone of voice, posture, and speech; thinking is slow, speech is sparse and voice volume is low. The patient may speak softly with a "flat" affect, looking down or away from you, and may be tearful. Sometimes a statement such as "You look sad" or "You look like all this is beginning to get you down" gives the patient an opportunity to talk about depressed feelings, thereby facilitating other more "medical" aspects of the history.

Some patients have endured such tragic events that you fear being overwhelmed with the sadness of it all. In such instances, it is appropriate to say that you, too, find the situation sad; in this way you make it clear to the patient that you are a fellow human being with feelings. In addition to this commonality, however, you are also a professional, and your feelings should be used constructively to help the patient. Here is an example that has both a feeling focus and a constructive focus. The patient is a 57-year-old woman who had coronary bypass surgery at the age of 53, followed 2 years later by a left radical mastectomy for aggressive carcinoma of the breast. She is now suffering from metastatic disease and is about to lose her health insurance coverage because her husband's business is failing and they can no longer afford the coverage.

Dr: A lot of bad things have happened to you. You must be a pretty strong person to have endured all this . . . How have you managed?

Pt: Well, I have my faith . . . and my family has been just wonderful to me.

Notice how the physician acknowledges the feeling content but, instead of getting deep into the tragedy, allows the patient to express her strength and her coping style. This technique serves the dual purpose of keeping both patient and physician from being overwhelmed.

Often the best follow-up questions are simple statements such as "Tell me more about these feelings" or "Tell me more about it," or the use of simple prompters and facilitators such as "Mm hmm" followed by silence to allow the patient to continue. Often this technique uncovers information vital to the diagnostic process:

Dr: You look sad. Is it about this chest pain you're having or something else?

Pt: I guess I am sad. My chest has been hurting all week. Well . . . see . . . I don't know if I can say it . . . I get all choked up . . . excuse me (trying to hold back tears). My mother died on Monday. Every time I think about her I get this choked-up feeling in here and it starts to hurt like my angina down into my arm.

Here the physician discovers the crucial connection between an exacerbation of the patient's angina and the recent death of the patient's mother.

Although perhaps more appropriate to a discussion of depression as an illness, no discussion of depression would be complete without considering questions to assess the depth of depression, particularly assessment of suicide risk. Some useful questions are:

- Do you get pretty discouraged (or blue)?
- What do you see for yourself in the future? How do you see the future?
- Do you ever feel that life isn't worth living? Or that you'd just as soon be dead? Or that you just can't go on?

And if answers to the above questions indicate a risk of suicide:

- Have you ever thought of hurting yourself? Of doing away with yourself? Of ending your life? Of suicide?
- Are you having any thoughts of hurting yourself? Of killing yourself?

- Did you ever think about how you would do it?

- What would happen to your family (parents, spouse, and so on) after you were dead?

It is important to give the patient time to answer these questions. Most patients are relieved to talk about feelings of suicide; such discussion does not put the idea of suicide into their heads. Here is an example of an assessment of suicide risk in a patient who is seeing an internist for follow-up of abdominal pain and asthma:

Dr: Last time I talked to you, you were feeling pretty bad.

Pt: You know, sometimes I scare myself.

Dr: You mean . . . have you ever tried to kill yourself?

Pt: Yeah.

Dr: How did you do it? How did you try?

Pt: Uh, I turned on the gas once.

Dr: What happened?

Pt: Somebody, they smelled the gas.

Dr: When was that?

Pt: That's not the first time I tried to kill myself. One time I climbed up on the bridge.

Dr: Uh hmm. What stopped you?

Pt: I don't know.

Dr: I'm glad you stopped. How are you feeling right now?

It is not uncommon that the need to assess suicide risk arises within the context of routine care for ordinary medical problems. Notice how this physician does not shy away from asking specific questions about past and current suicide intent. The physician also reaches out to the patient by sharing genuine happiness ("I'm glad you stopped") that the patient is still alive.

Denial

Denial is a common response to illness that most patients have, at least to some degree. It is the feeling that "This isn't really happening to me," "I can't believe it," or "That wasn't blood I saw in my bowel movement—at least, I don't think it was." In some patients the denial is strong enough that they either ignore or do not remember symptoms. Alternatively, patients may play down a worrisome symptom and report it as a trivial event: "I had a little pain in my chest, but it only lasted an hour." Only later do you find out that the pain was not only severe but also associated with nausea and sweating and a feeling of impending doom.

Whereas some patients play down the symptoms, others deny the emotional impact of a particular diagnosis or prognosis. At times, it is hard to tell the difference between denial and optimism, such as in the patient with a potentially lethal disease who smiles and says, "I know I can beat it." When patients accept bad news with apparent equanimity, it is difficult to know whether they are "handling it well" or denying some or all of the meaning of the diagnosis or prognosis. Denial can lead to serious delays in seeking care, but it is also a useful mechanism by which many patients cope with bad news. The clinician, therefore, should handle denial with circumspection and respect while trying to assess the patient's understanding of what is happening. Some useful techniques for doing this include:

- Accept denial as the patient's unique and current experience.

- Inform the patient gently and calmly that many people feel differently, including you. For example, you can say, "Most people feel very sad when they hear they have a serious illness," or "I guess I would be worried."

- Drop the subject if the patient is silent. The patient may come back to it, tentatively saying that once or twice he or she has felt as you described.

Consider this example of a young woman who came to the doctor for a "check-up." This was her first visit to this physician. On palpating the abdomen, the physician found a large mass which, on pelvic examination and subsequent ultrasound, proved to be an enormous uterine fibroid. The patient seemed unaware of its presence, despite the fact that the mass was the size of a 5-month pregnancy. When she was told that a hysterectomy might be necessary, she seemed unconcerned. The physician needed to find out if this 30-year-old woman who had not yet had children understood what a hysterectomy would mean to her, and was accepting that, or simply did not understand the implications of the surgery.

Dr: You don't seem very concerned at the idea of a hysterectomy.

Pt: Well, if I have to have it, that's it.

Dr: Do you know what a hysterectomy is?

Pt: Well, I guess that's when they take everything out.

Dr: Well, actually, it means the removal of the uterus or womb, that's where this fibroid is. Now this tumor is an overgrowth in the muscle, but even though it's not cancer, it may be impossible to remove without removing the uterus. Now your ovaries, which are the glands next to the uterus that make female hormones like estrogen, you've heard of estrogen? Okay, the ovaries would not be removed. (Draws picture.) They would stay, so your hormones would still work right.

Pt: But I still couldn't have babies.

Dr: That's right, you couldn't have babies. What do you think about that?

Pt: I don't know. I guess I never thought much about it, not being married and all, but I guess it hasn't really hit me yet. I'm more worried about the operation itself.

Notice how the physician gently probes the patient's knowledge and offers a clear explanation as to what will happen. The patient is not denying the outcome of the surgery but is, perhaps, delaying dealing with it pending resolution of her more immediate fears about the operation itself.

Patients' and Interviewers' Feelings About Each Other

The interaction between the interviewer and the patient may be highly charged with emotion. This relationship may bring out attitudes and behaviors reflecting either one's previous relationships. The sicker the patient, and the more helpless and dependent he or she is, the more likely it is that the patient's attitude toward the clinician will reflect a great deal of previously learned attitudes and experiences. Sometimes these attitudes are manifest in ways that appear totally irrational to the interviewer. For example, a patient who has had an angry, competitive relationship with his father may perceive a male physician as a powerful authority and may become antagonistic, sarcastic, and competitive, even though the physician has done nothing that would ordinarily elicit such a response. Similarly, female professionals may encounter seemingly irrational responses based on the patient's early experiences with being mothered. Although you may not be able to figure it out at the time, there is always a reason for what looks like irrational behavior.

Your interaction with the patient is, of course, two-sided; patients have feelings about you, and you most certainly have feelings about your patients. You may try to hide these feelings or even wonder if it is appropriate to have them. You will like some patients a lot and others less; there will probably be some that you actively dislike. Some will make you angry, and others you will dread. Some will make you laugh, and you will wonder whether it is "professional" to do so. You may even feel sexually attracted to certain patients and feel embarrassed or behave awkwardly.

The best approach to such feelings is first to identify and acknowledge them, at least to yourself. Think: How is the patient making me uncomfortable? And why? The answer to the "how" questions will allow you to identify behaviors in the patient that are helpful in your assessment. For example, ask yourself whether you dread seeing this patient because the individual makes too many demands on you. If so, the patient may be an "entitled demander" that we spoke of earlier and will require particular attention during your interview. Alternatively, perhaps you are uncomfortable with another patient who is depressed or dying; you are afraid that there is nothing you can do for the individual. Remember, this is your problem, not the patient's. You may want to share such feelings with helpful colleagues. As you become comfortable with these feelings, you will be able to share them with the patient and so improve his or her self-understanding. The opportunity to create a real connection with your patient can be the basis for a professional intimacy as you learn more about each other over time.

S U M M A R Y : Diagnosing and Treating the "Sick" Interview

Although we'd like all interviews with our patients to go well, sometimes our best efforts to apply basic skills go awry. When this happens, our relationship with the patient may be impaired, and, more pertinent to this text, our ability to get accurate and precise data is impaired: we may ascribe too much importance to one symptom, ascribe too little to another, or miss a vital one entirely. In this chapter, we have explored common sources of interviewing problems including interactive styles, somatization, and feelings. Although it is useful to discuss each as a distinct category, problems rarely present in pure form, and a number of common approaches are helpful to diagnose and treat the "sick" interview:

- View the problem as one involving the interaction itself as opposed to involving only the patient. All patients (and all interviewers) have personality styles and feelings; problems arise especially when there is a mismatched or exaggerated response by either party.

- Try to diagnose the problem. (Is this seemingly angry patient really depressed? Are these requests reasonable? Why not?)

- Observe the basics of good interviewing technique (open-ended questions, time for the patient to respond, use of summaries and interchangeable responses).

- Accept and respect the patient's feelings and coping style.

- Focus on good interactions, which, repeated over time, lead to productive relationships.

- Establish some control over the relationship, which means setting goals, limits, and guidelines. Remember that the patient wants some control over his or her frightening feelings and will appreciate a method to deal with them.

What can you do for yourself as you struggle with these difficult interactions? Somatizing patients, exaggerated personality styles, and certain feelings hit us in two vulnerable places. First, these patients defy the comfort of mind-body separation. They may present us with the unending conundrum of "when to say when"; after all, there is always the remote possibility that we have, indeed, missed an occult physical explanation for their symptoms. Second, these patients place a great deal of stress on our already fragile emotions. We may see them as oppositional, demanding, recalcitrant, perverse, frustrating, or futile. One difficult interaction or "dreaded patient" on the morning's schedule can sour your whole day.

A health-care professional who gets in touch with his or her own feelings and is able to discuss them with colleagues is much more likely to "survive" difficult interactions. One setting in which this can occur is a Balint group, a type of regular, small-group meeting named after the British psychiatrist Michael Balint.[7] In such a group, a number of clinicians and a psychiatrist or psychologist discuss the care of difficult patients and the difficult feelings such patients engender. Developing strategies for those times when you feel yourself reacting (often with too little sympathy but, at times, with too much) will help you maintain your empathic focus on the patient. These strategies will also be useful as you anticipate giving a patient bad news and as you deal with the dying patient, topics covered in the next chapter.

References

1. Kahana RJ, Bibring GL. Personality types in medical management. In: Zinberg NE. (Ed.) *Psychiatry and Medical Practice in a General Hospital.* New York, International Universities Press, 1964, pp. 108–123.
2. Groves JE. Taking care of the hateful patient. *N Engl J Med* 1978; 398:883–887.
3. Katon W, Ries RK, Kleinman A. A prospective DSM-III study of 100 somatization patients. *Compr Psychiatry* 1984; 25:305–314.
4. Block MR, Schulberg HC, Coulehan JL, et al. Recognition and characteristics of depression in primary care practice. *J Am Board Fam Pract* 1988; 1:91–97.
5. Coulehan JL, Schulberg HC, Block MR, et al. Symptom patterns of depression in ambulatory medical and psychiatric patients. *J Nerv Ment Dis* 1988; 176:284–288.
6. Lipkin M Jr. Psychiatry and medicine. In: Kaplan H, Sadock B. (Eds.) *Comprehensive Textbook of Psychiatry,* 5th ed. Baltimore, Williams & Wilkins, 1987.
7. Balint M. *The Doctor, His Patient and the Illness.* New York, International Universities Press, 1972.

Suggested Readings

American Psychiatric Association: Somatoform disorders In: *Diagnostic and Statistical Manual of Mental Disorders,* 4th ed. Washington, DC, American Psychiatric Association, 1994, pp. 445–469.

Barsky AJ, Klerman GL. Overview: Hypochondriasis, body complaints and somatic styles. *Am J Psychiatry* 1983; 140:273–282.

Billings JA, Stoeckle JD. *The Clinical Encounter*. Chicago, Yearbook Medical Publishers, 1989.

Callahan EJ, Bertakis KD, Rahman A, et al. The influence of depression on physician-patient interaction in primary care. *Fam Med* 1996; 28:346–351.

deGruy F, Columbia L, Dickinson P. Somatization disorder in a family practice. *J Fam Pract* 1987; 25:45–51.

deGruy F, Crider J, Hashimi DK, et al. Somatization disorder in a university hospital. *J Fam Pract* 1987; 25:579–584.

Escobar JI, Burnam MA, Karno M, et al. Somatization in the community. *Arch Gen Psychiatry* 1987; 44:713–718.

Quill TE. Recognizing and adjusting to barriers in doctor-patient communication. *Ann Intern Med* 1989; 111:51–57.

Shea SC. *Psychiatric Interviewing: The Art of Understanding*. Philadelphia, WB Saunders, 1988.

CHAPTER 11

Something New
and Dreadful

• • •

TELLING BAD NEWS

There was no deceiving himself: something new and dreadful
was happening to him, something of such vast importance that
nothing in his life could compare with it.

Leo Tolstoy, *The Death of Ivan Ilych*

Telling bad news is among the most difficult interpersonal situations that
clinicians encounter. The concept of honesty is a relatively new one in medicine; for example, as recently as the 1960s, most American physicians routinely misled cancer patients about their diagnosis and, especially, the prognosis of their condition. This paternalistic tradition was based on the belief
that the knowledge that they were suffering from a fatal illness would actually be harmful to many or most persons. These patients would lose all
hope of being cured, the argument went, thus damaging their quality of life
and perhaps even shortening their lives because of the loss of the "will to
live." The last 30 years have seen a remarkable reversal of these beliefs. We
now know that nearly all people desire to know their prognosis and that
such knowledge is far more helpful than harmful to them. Of equal importance is the development of greater respect for patient autonomy or self-
determination as a fundamental principle of medical ethics. We now have a
better appreciation of patient rights, especially the right to choose (or refuse)
treatment. This right demands that patients be given adequate information

about diagnosis and prognosis, as well as the risks and benefits of therapy. Thus, today it is standard practice in the United States for physicians to tell their patients bad news.

During the same period, another change has taken place. We have also tended to neglect some of the more positive features of the traditional image of caring for dying patients. In the past, when there was little that could be done to change the course of fatal illnesses, clinicians emphasized the caring aspects of their role; they could, at least, remain faithful, available, and supportive to dying patients and their families. Witness our traditional images of frequent house calls and bedside vigils. Now that medicine has enormous power to intervene, we focus almost exclusively on the technical aspects of what we can do for a patient: Can the cancer be cured? Will chemotherapy be beneficial? When the answer to all such questions is negative, we then conclude that the physician's role is finished. There is "nothing more" to do. The lack of technical potency makes clinicians feel uncomfortable, so we tend to minimize our interactions with the patient, rather than remaining available and using the therapeutic power of the clinician-patient relationship to provide physical and emotional support.

In this chapter we present an approach to telling bad news that develops from the basic interactive skills featured throughout this book. The first section examines and illustrates a series of personal and cultural barriers we must overcome in order to communicate bad news clearly and empathically. The second section outlines a skill-based approach to improving these difficult interactions. In the last part of the chapter, we take up the topic of advance directives and the way to incorporate discussion about advance directives into routine patient care.

BARRIERS TO COMMUNICATING BAD NEWS

Table 11–1 lists several psychologic and professional barriers that clinicians must overcome in order to communicate bad news in a clear and effective manner. In this section we describe and illustrate them, partly through the voices of patients.

TABLE 11–1 BARRIERS TO TELLING BAD NEWS

- Denying defeat: There is always a chance.
- Filtering the data: Professional language disguises the truth.
- Fear of diminishing hope: The patient needs the will to live.
- Keeping your distance: Feeling feelings is unprofessional.
- Disappearing: There is nothing I can do.

The Physician Delays: Denying Defeat

Given the wide array of available diagnostic tests and treatment options, it is perhaps natural that physicians tend to wait until the last possible minute to tell bad news. In a sense, they convince themselves the news is not really *that* bad—at least not *now*. After all, this argument goes, there are additional tests to be done. Perhaps these tests will show that the cancer has not yet metastasized. Why tell the patient the diagnosis before we have the whole picture? Why create useless anxiety? Alternatively, after cancer surgery a physician might ask himself or herself: "Why discuss the fact that we were unable to remove the whole tumor? Let's wait until the patient is stronger and better able to take the news."

This approach essentially denies the reality of terminal illness by postponing discussion about it simply because the physician lacks certain information about the prognosis. This form of denial obviously flounders on the shoals of respect for self-determination and the doctrine of informed consent: A patient cannot make informed choices about his or her care without knowing what the problem is.

The Physician Filters the Truth: Confusion Instead of Clarity

When clinicians do give bad news, they often do so obliquely or in a language that the patient doesn't understand, hiding behind disease-specific issues (e.g., the name of the cancer and what the treatment is) rather than addressing the patient's human concerns in simple, clear language. Alternatively, they may use vague language that is literally true ("The tumor isn't responding as well as we would like it to") but does not convey the meaning of the situation. The following example illustrates this type of miscommunication[1]:

Dr: Your mother's condition is deteriorating, and we don't expect her to do too well.

Family: Thank you, doctor, we know you are doing your best.

Dr: Well, so far we've been able to keep her blood pressure up with pressors.

Family: That's good, isn't it? At least the blood pressure isn't a problem. (Physician leaves)

Family to each other: Thank goodness, he didn't say she's dying.

The use of complex descriptions about *what can be done* to disguise honest discussion about *what it all means* is probably the most common form of miscommunication in caring for dying patients. This type of interchange is illustrated in Leo Tolstoy's *The Death of Ivan Ilych*[2] when Ivan Ilych realizes that "something new and dreadful was happening to him, something of such vast importance that nothing in his life could compare with it" (p. 80). His physician blathers on about technical details, such as telling him the problem is a "floating kidney" and then describing in detail just how it became detached and what might be done about it. Later, Ivan Ilych goes to another physician who tells him that the problem is "a tiny little thing in the caecum" and then proceeds to describe what must be done: "Stimulate the energy of one organ, depress the activity of another" (p. 87). But none of the physicians addresses the most important issue: "To Ivan Ilych only one question mattered: was his condition serious or not?" (p. 75).

In an essay describing his recovery from a devastating stroke, Robert McCrum wrote about his physicians' retreat into vague language: ". . . The experts took refuge in a studied vagueness—'probably' I'd be fit in 'about a year'; after six months, it would be 'fairly clear' how much movement would return to my left side; then 'perhaps' my arm would become 'useful.'"[3] Functional outcome after a stroke is, of course, uncertain. Yet there is an enormous difference between sharing this uncertainty with the patient in an interactive and constructive way and relying on broad terms or qualifiers to create a "studied vagueness."

A contemporary example of medical gobbledygook, combined with a large dose of emotional detachment, is illustrated in Evan Handler's *Time on Fire*. Evan Handler, a young New York actor, was admitted to a world-famous cancer hospital for treatment of his acute leukemia. He recalls overhearing his hospital roommate's physicians on rounds: "On the far side of the curtain they would gruffly lay out absolutely horrifying scenarios and treatment plans in very complex language, then leave and joke and laugh their way down the hall."[4] (p. 26). In a research study of how bad news was communicated to the parents of pediatric patients, one mother reported, "I don't want them to unnecessarily scare the hell out of me—but I *hate* the feeling of being in the dark. Especially when a new problem appears with a medical name a mile long, I don't know the 'right' questions to ask."[5] (Her 4-year-old child suffered from cerebral palsy.) Like the other examples in this section, these behaviors illustrate the use of words to create or maintain distance, rather than to facilitate genuine communication.

The Physician Wills to Live: Not Destroying Hope

This dynamic is well-characterized by the Yale surgeon Sherwin Nuland in his best-selling book, *How We Die*: "Too often physicians misunderstand the ingredients of hope, thinking it refers only to cure or remission. They feel it necessary to transmit to a cancer-ridden patient by inference if not by actual statement, the erroneous assumption that it is still possible to attain months if not years of symptom-free life. When an otherwise totally honest and beneficent physician is asked why he does this, his answer is likely to be some variation of, 'Because I didn't want to take away his only hope.'" (p. 223).[6]

In the past, physicians justified their reluctance to "tell it like it is" because they thought the truth would harm the patient by taking away all hope and perhaps causing a loss of the will to live. It seemed reasonable then that truthfulness was often at odds with the Hippocratic dictum, "Help, or at least do no harm." We now know this in most cases to be false, yet it is still difficult, when faced with a real patient in a real situation, not to think that perhaps the truth should be watered down or delayed in *this* particular case. There is almost a sense in which the better the relationship we have with a patient, the more difficult it might be to avoid the "loss-of-hope fallacy." If a patient is important to us, it is easy to imagine many ways in which bad news might cause him or her harm. Alternatively, physicians who stick to the technical aspects of medicine might have an easier time of it—if you can't imagine a person's life narrative, psychologic harm remains simply an abstract concept rather than a real concern. Dr. Nuland illustrates precisely this dynamic when he describes his own intervention in his brother's terminal illness. Even though he was quite aware that both he and his brother's physicians should be completely truthful about the dismal prognosis, "I did exactly what I warned others against" (p. 226). Because he loved his brother so much, he confused the hopelessness of curing or ameliorating his metastatic colon cancer with human hopelessness. Not wanting his brother to face the latter, Nuland orchestrated deceptive options, encouraging his brother's belief that additional treatment might arrest the tumor.[6]

The Physician Is Detached: Maintaining Distance

Health-care professionals also have difficulty dealing with the emotional aspects of talking about dying and death. They may not want to confront their own feelings about dying. They may be frightened by the patient's, or a family member's, potentially strong emotional response to the news, and by continuing emotional involvement. They may feel awkward and not know what to say. Physicians who are extraordinarily skillful at detached, technical aspects of medicine may at the same time be very insecure in dealing with sensitive interpersonal relationships. This leads dying patients to feel emotionally abandoned.

In *Intoxicated by My Illness*, a posthumous collection of essays about his experience as a cancer patient, the literary critic Anatole Broyard wrote about the tendency of his physicians to remain detached: "(Some) doctors give you a generic, unfocused gaze. They look at you panoramically. They don't see you in focus . . . If he could gaze directly at the patient, the doctor's work would be more gratifying. Why bother with sick people, why try to save them, if they're not worth acknowledging? When a doctor refuses to acknowledge a patient, he is, in effect, abandoning him to his illness" (p. 50).[7]

Broyard also went on to describe what he desired in a physician treating him during terminal illness—not necessarily a close friend or hand-holder, but someone who was carefully observant, emotionally honest, and insightful: "Now that I know I have cancer of the prostate, the lymph nodes, and part of my skeleton, what *do* I want in a doctor? I would say that I want one who is a close reader of illness and a good critic of medicine . . . " (p. 40).[7] He wanted most of all to be viewed as a fellow human being, not just a face in a bed or across a desk: "I would like my doctor to understand that beneath my surface cheerfulness, I feel . . . 'the panic inherent in creation' and 'the suction of infinity' " (p. 42).[7]

Detachment may be manifested by inappropriate, as well as absent, emotional responses. Some clinicians conceal their detachment behind a facade of exaggerated cheerfulness or chumminess. These fake feelings may be a medical manifestation of our superficial "Have a good day" culture. For example, the writer Marjorie Gross described how her physician told her she had ovarian cancer: "So I'm sitting in the doctor's office, he walks in, just tells me straight out, 'I was right—it's ovarian cancer, so I win. Pay up.' And I say, 'Oh, no, you're not gonna hold me to that, are you?' And he says, 'Hey, a bet's a bet' " (p. 54).[8]

The Physician Vanishes: Disappearing

When patients become terminally ill, they sometimes find that their physicians have performed a vanishing act. There are a number of reasons for this. First, if a clinician is oriented toward using office visits only for "medical indications," he or she might feel there is no justification for frequent visits—after all, the patient is not on "active" treatment. Likewise, the hospital physician may have plenty of complicated decisions to make on rounds and not feel he or she has the time to spend "socializing" in a dying patient's room. Second, terminally ill patients may have difficulty getting around; since house calls are rare nowadays, these patients may find it physically difficult to see their physicians. Finally, many physicians find it emotionally difficult to care for dying patients. Oriented toward aggressive therapy and attempts to cure, they are very uncomfortable with the maxim, "Don't just do something; sit there." Thus, they either tell the patient explicitly, or communicate implicitly, "There is nothing more I can do."

During the long and devastating ordeal of his treatment for acute leukemia, Evan Handler found a few physicians who were able to overcome these barriers and avoid disappearing, either physically or emotionally. He describes one of them in the following paragraph: "Dr. Gee chatted easily with me, in a soothing voice, before moving on to the medical matters at hand. Even after the transition to business had occurred, I found his demeanor to be exquisitely sensitive to the fact that he had come into the temporary home of another individual. Dr. Gee explained precisely what type of examination he *hoped* to perform, rather than planned to. He asked me how I felt about everything he proposed. Dr. Gee asked me to let him know if there were any areas that I was especially apprehensive about having examined. . . . Timothy Gee, from the moment he entered the room, made no assumption of superiority and held no illusions that asserting it might simplify his assignment." (p. 175).[4]

In the next section we analyze skills like those of Dr. Gee in more detail.

EMPATHY AND INTERACTION IN TELLING BAD NEWS

Setting the Stage

The first step in effectively communicating bad news (Table 11–2) is to prepare yourself for the encounter and select an appropriate setting. In the hospital this means choosing a relatively quiet time to sit by the patient's bed, a time when you don't have to jump up and finish rounds or answer pages. Some patients prefer the presence of a spouse or other family members; others prefer to receive the news on their own. The old practice of informing the patient's family first—and then deciding whether the patient himself or herself should be told—is clearly disrespectful and paternalistic. It is also a serious breach of physician-patient confidentiality. When a patient is elderly or very ill, it often seems natural to speak with a family member first about diagnosis or prognosis. In some such cases this may be appropriate because it is clearly consistent with the patient's wishes. However, it should also be made clear that the patient has a right to know. If family members request your collusion in hiding the news from the patient (e.g.,

---

TABLE 11–2 COMMUNICATING BAD NEWS IN THE CLINICAL SETTING

Setting the Stage
- Choose a quiet setting
- Give the news in person, not by phone
- Allocate adequate time for discussion

Telling the News
- Use simple, clear language
- Avoid the temptation to minimize the problem
- Assess the patient's emotional state
- Express sorrow for the patient's situation

Continuing the Interview
- Assess how the patient feels after receiving the news
- Reassure the patient of your continued availability
- Communicate a plan for care if not cure

for cultural reasons), you must explore the options thoroughly and perhaps request help from others who are more familiar with the patient's cultural background (see Chap. 14) before agreeing to mask the truth. Only if the patient has limited or absent decision-making capacity will you will have to conduct the conversation with the patient's surrogate and other family members.

Giving bad news over the phone is almost always a bad decision. Consider the following example:[9]

Dr: [speaking to the patient by telephone] The bad news is that you have a brain tumor. The good news is that we think it's a meningioma, which means it'll be easy for us to get to.

Pt: [long pause] What, what are you saying? . . . I don't know what you mean.

Dr: I mean it's a probably a benign tumor on the outside of your brain, so we can remove it by surgery.

Pt: Uh . . . I don't know what to say. . . . Can I come in and talk with you about this?

Dr: Okay, yes, we can do that. Call Judy. Let's make an appointment for next Tuesday.

In this case the physician's flip "good news/bad news" opening demonstrates his insensitivity to the human dimension of his message. He seems to believe that having a meningioma is a wonderful opportunity for the patient, certainly nothing to become upset about. When the patient requests a meeting, this physician blithely suggests a future appointment and asks the patient herself to set it up ("Call Judy"). He has neither allowed adequate time for discussion of the news today—after all, the patient can't suspend her feelings until next week—nor assessed the patient's emotional state to determine what needs to be done right now.

How could this situation have been handled better? First, the physician or his office could have called to arrange a prompt appointment to discuss the test results. Second, as we discuss in the next section, he could have approached the topic in a direct and emotionally appropriate manner without minimizing the issue or hiding behind euphemisms.

Telling the News

It is usually good to preface your remarks with a clear statement like, "I'm afraid I have bad news." The patient will already know by your behaviors (e.g., an intake of breath, an uncharacteristic hesitation) that something is wrong. It is best to avoid the natural temptation to tip-toe up to the main point by beginning with small talk or side issues. You will be better able to help the patient by spending the entire time explaining the situation, answering the patient's questions, and providing emotional support. There is also a risk that, if you begin slowly, you will end up minimizing the problem (see Table 11–2) by stopping at half-truths or leaving important facts unexplained. Here is an example of a physician beginning to tell bad news in a clear, straightforward way:[10]

Dr: Good morning, Mr. Lee. How are you feeling today?

Pt: Better than I did a week ago.

Dr: I'm glad of that. We have some very serious matters to discuss regarding your health. Do you feel ready for this discussion?

Pt: Well, I want to know. I'll try to be ready

Dr: It's hard to ever be ready for bad news. This is not easy. I need to let you know that we got the results of your test back. . . . As we had feared, the lump is a malignant tumor, cancer.

In this case the physician moves almost directly from "We have some very serious matters to discuss . . . " to "It's hard to ever be ready for bad news." Her one intervening question is, "Do you feel ready for this discussion?" An important aspect of this type of encounter is assessing the patient's emotional state, both directly by specific questions and indirectly through paralanguage and nonverbal cues (see Chap. 2). The clinician should acknowledge the difficulty of the situation and adjust the pace and form of the presentation based on an assessment of the patient's emotional needs. It is appropriate to express sorrow for the patient's pain. This may involve not only verbal expressions of concern but also nonverbal evidence of solidarity, such as maintaining good eye contact, reaching out and touching the patient's hand or sleeve, or even shedding a tear.

Continuing the Interview

As the interview progresses, it is important for the clinician to monitor both the patient's understanding of the information and his or her emotional response to the news. With regard to understanding, patients who have just received bad news are unlikely to remember complex information regarding diagnostic strategies or treatment options.[11] Thus, it is usually best to stick to the major points, reiterate them, offer to answer questions, and arrange for your continued availability, including a prompt follow-up appointment. Often, however, one or more specific tasks need to be done relatively quickly, such as further diagnostic studies to delineate the extent of disease, or urgent radiation therapy in the case of threatened spinal cord compression. In such cases, it may be necessary to discuss technical issues at the same time you are breaking the bad news. To help facilitate the patient's retention of information, follow the guidelines suggested in Chapter 9 (p. 170, Table 9–3). Other useful suggestions to consider include:

- If the patient agrees, encourage at least one other family member to participate in the interview.
- Illustrate your major points with charts and drawings.
- Make an audiotape of the interview for the patient to keep and review at home.
- If available, lend the patient videotapes that describe the condition and relevant tests or treatments.

At all stages of the interview, check the patient's understanding and invite questions. At the end, summarize and recheck.

Patients' emotional responses may vary greatly. Some may be very calm and cool, focusing entirely on technical details. This reaction (or lack of reaction) is likely to relieve the anxious physician, who then might conclude that his or her patient is coping exceptionally well. However, extreme calmness suggests that the person either hasn't really understood the news, or hasn't emotionally "connected" with it. It might be useful for the physician to draw attention to this lack of response, "I notice you are taking this situation very calmly, but in my experience many people react differently."

Other patients might display anger and hostility. One of the authors cared for a middle-aged man who had, in a period of weeks, developed facial flushing, shortness of breath when lying down, and other symptoms of the superior vena cava syndrome. This indicated that something (e.g., a tumor) was compromising the venous return to the heart from the upper part of his body. Because it took 2 weeks to accomplish the diagnostic studies and arrange a mediastinoscopy, which ultimately revealed that he had non-Hodgkin's lymphoma, the patient responded to the news with angry comments about what he perceived to be a delay in diagnosis. Why hadn't we acted quicker? Why wasn't the hospital more efficient? In such cases it is always best to acknowledge the anger without minimizing it or trying to explain it away. You might say, "I know this is upsetting news. I understand your feelings and I do want to help." Some patients will combine anger with denial, challenging the diagnosis or demanding a second opinion. Again, the clinician should acknowledge the shocking nature of the news and support the patient in obtaining another opinion ("I think that's a good idea, do you have someone in mind?") if he or she so desires.

This chapter focuses on "breaking" bad news and its immediate aftermath. Telling bad news is not an isolated event; it is a process that may extend over several visits and several conversations. In many cases the bad news ushers in a period of intensive therapy that leads to remission or cure.

In other cases, however, therapy to alter the course of the disease will be ineffective and treatment should be directed to symptom relief. The care of terminally ill patients presents continuing difficulties for physicians. The fewer the "medical" options available, the more difficult it is to overcome the barriers of avoidance, partial truth, emotional distance, and so forth, which prevent us from facing the patient. In the interview, it is important to communicate a plan for continued care, even when remission or cure is impossible. This plan should be specific to the patient's needs and renewed as appropriate at each contact; for example, you might say,

- "No matter what happens, I'll do my best to see this through with you . . . I won't abandon you."
- "I want you to know I'll continue to be available. You can always call me if you have questions or problems . . . I'll get back to you."
- "My goal is for you to be as comfortable and functional as possible. We have good medications to help us do that. But you and I have to work together."

ADVANCE DIRECTIVES

An advance directive is a written statement ("living will") or an explicit arrangement with another person (health-care proxy or durable power of attorney) that allows a patient's wishes regarding treatment to be honored, even when the patient loses his or her decision-making capacity. The Patient Self-Determination Act is a Federal law requiring that patients be informed about advance directives upon admission to acute-care hospitals and some chronic-care facilities. The idea, of course, is to give patients the opportunity to consider their own treatment objectives and express them, or to appoint a surrogate decision-maker prior to the possibility of losing their capacity during that hospitalization or a subsequent one. When a patient is admitted to the hospital, however, he or she is generally not physically or psychologically well-prepared for a reasoned discussion about health-care choices near the end of life. Likewise, physicians and other health professionals dealing with a patient's acute overwhelming illness are not likely to set a high priority on explaining advance directives and their meaning. **Thus, the best time to interview patients regarding advance directives is during their ongoing outpatient care, particularly in the primary-care setting.**

With whom should you raise the topic of advance directives? First, it is useful to include a question about whether or not a patient has a "living will" or has designated a health-care proxy in every initial medical history on a new adult patient. If you use a structured questionnaire as a method of obtaining some initial data (see Chap. 12), these questions may be included on the questionnaire. Because the patient profile should include information about the person's health beliefs and values, the existence and character of an advance directive fits appropriately in that segment of the medical history.

Second, you should further explore the topic of advance directives with patients who have serious chronic or terminal illnesses. An important component of caring for such patients is a thorough discussion of their beliefs and values about life-sustaining treatment under various circumstances. The patient should receive information about written advance directives and health-care proxies, with particular emphasis on the appropriate legal mechanism in your state. Written information in the required forms should also be available in the office.

When initiating a discussion of advance directives, set the stage by giving a clear statement of the issue rather than making any assumptions about the patient's knowledge or asking pointed questions about treatment. Here is how one physician asked a patient about end-of-life-decisions:

Dr: Now we need to talk about living wills. You ought to consider signing a living will because if you become incompetent later in this illness, we need to know what you would want us to do, let's say, if we had to put you on a breathing machine.

This physician assumed that the patient would know what "living will" and "incompetent" mean. He failed to explain them or put them in perspective. A second physician also failed to "set the stage" well:

Dr: As I said, there is nothing more we can do to stop the disease from progressing, so we are going to be faced with some tough questions sooner or later. For example, if your heart stops, would you like us to do what we can to try to start it up again?

This physician immediately jumped to a very specific question about cardiopulmonary resuscitation. In addition, she began on the very negative note of, "There is nothing more we can do . . . "

A third physician did a better job of setting the stage for the discussion of advance directives:

Dr: Now we need to talk about what kinds of treatment decisions you would like somebody to make for you if you are no longer able to make your own decisions. What I'm thinking about is something we call a living will or a health-care proxy. You've probably heard about living wills. They are written statements that tell us what you would like us to do or not to do, let's say, if your illness reaches the point where we have to put you on a breathing machine and there is no hope that you will recover. A health proxy is just a person whom you designate now to speak for you and to make all your medical decisions for you if you become so ill you can't make your own choices. Lots of people have both living wills and health-care proxies. Would you like to discuss more about this now?

This physician was careful not only to set the stage for discussing the issue but also to allow the patient to decide whether the discussion should continue at that point. She was explicit about the meaning of living wills and health-care proxies and indicated that they are not incompatible. Likewise, she did not frame her reference to "breathing machine" in such a way as to make it a leading question. The exchange might continue in this way:

Pt: I don't know, I've heard about living wills, but I am not sure I know enough about them.

Dr: Well, I can give you a brochure that I think will answer a lot of your questions about living wills, and also it tells you about designating someone to make decisions for you. I can also give you the form for designating a proxy, so you can see what it looks like.

Pt: OK, doctor, but . . . I don't know, talking about this makes me feel like it's all over, you know, like there's no hope . . .

Dr: I can understand how you feel that, but it really means nothing of the sort. There's a lot we can do for you and you can do for yourself.. And you and I will work together on this. I'll respect your decisions every step of the way. That's really why I bring the issue up now . . . to make sure that we can continue respecting your choices and values if something happens that you can't tell us at the time. I guess you could call it a type of preventive medicine.

A major point in this dialogue is the physician's attempt to diffuse the understandable anxiety patients often have when confronted with the issue of advance directives. In this case, she makes sure that the patient understands that he is not "signing over" his participation in decision-making but rather is extending his participation beyond the point where it would normally end. Unlike the physician in the second example earlier, this clinician is also alleviating the patient's feeling that "Living will equals nothing-more-we-can-do."

S U M M A R Y : Communicating Bad News

We began this chapter by exploring five barriers to communicating bad news to patients (see Table 11–1). Health-care professionals tend to deny to themselves that the situation is as bad as it is and, therefore, delay telling the news; they use vague or complicated language; they believe that patients will lose hope if they know the truth about their prognosis; they become emotionally distant; and, finally, they disappear. To provide good care for terminally ill patients, these barriers must be overcome.

Before telling bad news, the clinician should set the stage by providing a comfortable environment and allowing sufficient time. It is usually best to begin with a direct statement like "I'm afraid I have bad news to tell you." Verbal and nonverbal expressions of sorrow and support are appropriate. As the interview progresses, the clinician should monitor the patient's understanding and emotional response, realizing that it is difficult for persons to "take in" and process so much significant information at once. Good continuing care for the critically ill and dying patient demands that the physician be both emotionally and physically accessible.

Advance directives help ensure that patients' wishes are respected, even if they lose decision-making capacity. A question about a living will or health-care proxy should be part of every initial medical interview. The topic of advance directives should be explored further with patients who suffer from serious chronic or terminal illness. The subject requires a direct and clear explanation, followed by willingness to answer questions and provide emotional support.

References

1. Campbell ML. Breaking bad news to patients. *JAMA* 1994; 271:1052.
2. Tolstoy L. *The Death of Ivan Ilych*. New York, Bantam Books, 1981.
3. McCrum R. My old and new lives. *The New Yorker*, May 27, 1996.
4. Handler E, *Time on Fire: My Comedy of Terrors*. Boston, Little, Brown, 1996.
5. Sharpe MC, Strauss RP, Lorch SC. Communicating medical bad news: Parents' experiences and preferences. *J Pediatr* 1992; 121:539–546.
6. Nuland SB. *How We Die*. New York, Alfred A. Knopf, 1994, p. 223.
7. Broyard A. *Intoxicated by My Illness*. New York, Clarkson Potter Publishers, 1992.

8. Gross M. Cancer becomes me. *The New Yorker*, April 15, 1996, pp. 54–55.
9. Lind SE, Good M, Seidel S, Csordas T, Good BJ. Telling the diagnosis of cancer. *J Clin Oncol* 1989; 7:583–589.
10. Miranda J, Brody RV. Communicating bad news. *West J Med* 1992; 156:83–85.
11. Block MR. The bad news. *JAMA* 1987; 257:2952.

Suggested Reading

Kaye P. *Symptom Control in Hospice and Palliative Care*. Essex, CT, Hospice Education Institute, 1994.

CHAPTER 12

The Quiz-Docs
Will Catch You

• • •

QUESTIONNAIRES AND COMPUTERS

And if you're the type that gets finicky-finick

At this point you'll try to get out of that clinic.

But they will outwit you as quick as a winick!

The Quiz-Docs will catch you!

They'll start questionnairing!

They'll ask you, point blank, how your parts are all faring.

Dr. Seuss, *You're Only Old Once*

Simple questions with "yes" or "no" answers can be useful in many parts of the medical interview, such as in the review of systems or in the delineation of certain characteristics of a symptom. As clinicians progress through the interview, they often use such **focused questioning** when building a case for a certain diagnosis; in other words, they ask whether a specific symptom is present (yes or no) in order to lend support for (confirm) or weigh against (dis-confirm) one or more specific diagnoses being considered. Since this sort of questioning is in some ways analogous to a branching protocol, physicians have for some time been interested in the possibility of using structured questionnaires, computer-generated protocols, or artificial intelligence programs to assist in taking the medical history. This process probably began

227

in the late 1940s with a comprehensive printed list of symptoms called the Cornell Medical Index. Currently, it includes a wide array of sophisticated instruments and interactive computer programs. In this chapter we briefly survey the uses of questionnaires and computer applications as adjuncts to the medical interview, especially with regard to medical history taking.

USES OF QUESTIONNAIRES

Questionnaires as Reminders

Some physicians ask new patients to complete standardized history forms or checklists before the patient's first appointment. Although questionnaires cannot replace talking with patients as a source of diagnostic information, carefully selected instruments can supplement the medical interview in two important ways. First, the process of thinking through a series of questions may refresh a patient's memory and focus his or her attention so that, ultimately, the interview yields a more complete narrative of the patient's medical history. This phenomenon is similar to the effect of repeated medical interviews; by the second or third time around, the patient may have constructed a more thoughtful narrative. An additional benefit is that, with a completed questionnaire at his or her disposal, the interviewer can focus the questioning more efficiently and "zero in" on particular problems or symptoms. Thus, checklists serve as useful reference points for discussion of past medical history, family history, and review of systems.

The review of systems is quite adaptable to a checklist approach (see Chap. 6). In this case, extensive and detailed checklists are very sensitive; that is, they are unlikely to miss any important symptoms. No false negatives can slip through the net, provided the patient understands the written questions. However, such checklists are not very specific; that is, many trivial symptoms that are unrelated to disease will surface, especially if the patient is thoughtful and complete in responding to the instructions. Patients may acknowledge a wide array of mild, intermittent, or transient symptoms, and the form itself may not permit an assessment of severity or level of patient concern. Thus, a symptom checklist may yield many false-positive symptoms; the clinician, then, must use the subsequent interview to explore each positive response, attempting to ascertain its clinical importance.

Case Finding by Questionnaire

The second important role of questionnaires in medical interviewing is their use as diagnostic aids or **case-finding** instruments. Some questionnaires have been designed to identify persons at high risk for certain disorders such as depression (e.g., the Beck Depression Inventory [BDI],* Inventory to Diag-

---

* Aaron T. Beck, copyright 1978, Center for Cognitive Therapy, 133 S. 36th St., Room 602, Philadelphia PA 19104.

nose Depression [IDD],[1] or Self-Rating Depression Scale [SDS][2]), alcohol abuse (e.g., the Michigan Alcoholism Screening Test [MAST][3]), or mental disorders in primary care (e.g., the PRIME-MD[4]). These are relatively short lists of questions structured so that either patients or clinicians can complete them in a few minutes.

Sometimes these instruments are called "screening tests" because, as with a traditional screening test, if a patient scores above a specified cutoff point, the clinician is expected to undertake a more complete diagnostic evaluation. These questionnaires are not, however, true screening tests. Routine blood pressure determination, serum cholesterol, mammography, cervical smears for cytology, sigmoidoscopy, and stool tests for occult blood are all widely used in primary medical care to screen for asymptomatic disease. One of the requirements for an effective screening test is that it identify patients whose disease is in a preclinical or asymptomatic phase, when early treatment can potentially prevent the full-blown clinical syndrome and its complications. Certain parts of the medical history are actually screening tests in this sense. For example, knowledge of cardiac risk factors is important in predicting and attempting to prevent heart disease. Thus, a risk factor profile is a screening test, analogous to a blood pressure check or a cholesterol determination. The patient's family history of heart disease, smoking habits, and exercise profile are all important screening data. In the same sense, any part of the medical history that relates to the risk of developing a disease or to the detection of an asymptomatic disease, rather than to the presence of an established disease, can be considered a screening test.

Unlike true screening tests, instruments like the BDI, IDD, and SDS rely on the fact that characteristic symptoms are already present. They simply direct the clinician's attention to a possible diagnosis—in this case, clinical depression—by assigning quantitative weight to a cluster of symptoms. This characteristic makes them case-finding instruments rather than screening instruments.

Questionnaires for Psychiatric Disorders

Case-finding questionnaires have been developed primarily for psychiatric disorders; this is understandable since most psychiatric disorders are, in fact, defined by the presence of a certain constellation of symptoms and behaviors. Diagnosis relies almost entirely on a thorough interview. Neither scans, blood tests, nor biopsies can serve as diagnostic clinchers. These questionnaires can be useful in interviewing medical patients because psychiatric conditions occur frequently in medical patients and physicians often fail to diagnose them correctly. Questionnaire scores might assist physicians in suspecting a condition and then making the proper diagnosis.

Depression is a prime example. Of all patients seen in primary medical care settings, 6 to 9 percent suffer from a major depressive disorder (approximately the same prevalence as hypertension),[5] and another large group experience other variants of depression. Yet less than half of all depressed patients are accurately diagnosed, and even fewer receive appropriate treatment. Why? Several factors may contribute. Medical physicians look first to physical illness and consider the possibility of a psychiatric disorder only after somatic disease is thoroughly ruled out. Physicians often do not understand how common depression is and how much morbidity—including physical morbidity—it may cause. They may be unaware that depression usually includes somatic or vegetative symptoms (e.g., fatigue, weight loss, sleep disorder, or difficulty with memory and concentration). Moreover, they may not be familiar with proper methods of treatment for depression. In some cases, clinicians may recognize the presence of depression but withhold formal diagnosis because they believe a psychiatric disorder stigmatizes the patient.

TABLE 12–1   SELF-RATING DEPRESSION SCALE (SDS)

Below are 20 statements. Please rate each using the following scale: 1 = none or a little of the time; 2 = some of the time; 3 = good part of the time; 4 = most or all of the time.

Please record your rating in the space to the left of each item.

_____ 1. I feel down-hearted, blue, and sad.

_____ 2. Morning is when I feel the best.

_____ 3. I have crying spells or feel like it.

_____ 4. I have trouble sleeping through the night.

_____ 5. I eat as much as I used to.

_____ 6. I enjoy looking at, talking to, and being with attractive women/men.

_____ 7. I notice that I am losing weight.

_____ 8. I have trouble with constipation.

_____ 9. My heart beats faster than usual.

_____ 10. I get tired for no reason.

_____ 11. My mind is as clear as it used to be.

_____ 12. I find it easy to do the things I used to.

_____ 13. I am restless and can't keep still.

_____ 14. I feel hopeful about the future.

_____ 15. I am more irritable than usual.

_____ 16. I find it easy to make decisions.

_____ 17. I feel that I am useful and needed.

_____ 18. My life is pretty full.

_____ 19. I feel that others would be better off if I were dead.

_____ 20. I still enjoy the things I used to do.

SOURCE: From Zung WK. A self-rating depression scale. *Arch Gen Psychiatry* 1965; 12:63–70. Copyright 1965, American Medical Association. Reprinted with permission.

Table 12–1 presents the SDS, a frequently used depression questionnaire. The SDS has a positive predictive value of 40 to 75 percent.[5] Because the predictive value depends partly on prior probability, a positive SDS result in a patient with a high risk of depression would have a higher predictive value than a positive result in a low-risk patient. Some examples of high-risk patients include persons with chronic disease, those who have unexplained physical symptoms, and those with a prior history of depression. The IDD and PRIME-MD are more recently developed questionnaires that are based on explicit diagnostic criteria for depression and other psychiatric disorders from the *Diagnostic and Statistical Manual of Psychiatric Disorders*, 4th Edition (*DSM-IV*).[1,4] While the IDD is amenable to patient self-report, the PRIME-MD is designed to be administered as a brief structured interview by a clinician. Positive results on these two instruments are very highly correlated with the presence of clinically important psychiatric diagnoses.

Table 12–2 presents the MAST, a 25-item questionnaire that focuses on abnormal drinking behavior as well as its social, legal, and health consequences. A score of 5 indicates a very high probability of alcohol abuse or dependence. Although this questionnaire is fairly long, much of the diagnostic information it yields can be obtained by using small subsets of MAST questions. For example, in one study the two questions, "Have you ever had a drinking problem?" and "Was your last drink within the last 24 hours?"—when combined—had a positive predictive value for alcoholism of 69 percent and a negative predictive value of 98 percent.[6] In other words, if the patient answers both question in the affirmative, there is better than two chances in three that he or she has a drinking problem; those who answer both questions in the negative have almost no chance of having a drinking problem.

Four questions have been widely used in the primary care setting to help identify patients with alcohol problems. These are the so-called **CAGE questions:**

- Have you ever felt you ought to Cut down on your drinking?
- Have people Annoyed you by criticizing your drinking?
- Have you ever felt bad or Guilty about your drinking?
- Have you ever had a drink first thing in the morning (Eye opener) to steady your nerves or get rid of a hangover?

If all answers are negative, alcohol abuse or dependence can be ruled out. If one or more are positive, the physician is sensitized to explore further the role of alcohol in the patient's life.

A third questionnaire is also useful in assessing the probability of alcohol abuse (Table 12–3), especially when interviewing patients in an emer-

TABLE 12–2 MICHIGAN ALCOHOLISM SCREENING TEST (MAST) QUESTIONNAIRE

Question	Points
1. Do you feel you are a normal drinker?	2
2. Have you ever awakened the morning after some drinking the night before and found that you could not remember a part of the evening before?	2
3. Does your spouse (or parents) ever worry or complain about your drinking?	1
4. Can you stop drinking without a struggle after one or two drinks?	2
5. Do you ever feel bad about your drinking?	1
6. Do friends or relatives think you are a normal drinker?	1
7. Do you ever try to limit your drinking to certain times of the day or to certain places?	0
8. Are you always able to stop drinking when you want to?	2
9. Have you ever attended a meeting of Alcoholics Anonymous (AA)?	5
10. Have you gotten into fights when drinking?	1
11. Has drinking ever created problems with you and your spouse?	2
12. Has your spouse (or other family member) ever gone to anyone for help about your drinking?	2
13. Have you ever lost friends or girlfriends or boyfriends because of drinking?	2
14. Have you ever gotten into trouble at work because of drinking?	2
15. Have you ever lost a job because of drinking?	2
16. Have you ever neglected your obligations, your family, or your work for two or more days in a row because you were drinking?	2
17. Do you ever drink before noon?	1
18. Have you ever been told you have liver trouble? Cirrhosis?	2
19. Have you ever had delirium tremens (DTs), severe shaking, heard voices, or seen things that were not there after heavy drinking?	2
20. Have you ever gone to anyone for help about your drinking?	5
21. Have you ever been in a hospital because of drinking?	5
22. Have you ever been a patient in a psychiatric hospital or on a psychiatric ward of a general hospital where drinking was part of the problem?	2
23. Have you ever been seen at a psychiatric or mental health clinic or gone to a doctor, social worker, or clergyman for help with an emotional problem in which drinking played a part?	2
24. Have you ever been arrested, even for a few hours, because of drunk behavior?	2
25. Have you ever been arrested for drunk driving or driving after drinking?	2

Score points for negative answers to questions 1, 4, 6, and 8 and positive answers to all other questions. A score of 5 or more points is highly suggestive of alcohol abuse.

SOURCE: From Selzer ML. The Michigan Alcoholism Screening Test: The quest for a new diagnostic instrument. *Am J Psychiatry* 127, 1653–1658, 1971. Copyright 1971, the American Psychiatric Association. Reprinted by permission.

TABLE 12–3 TRAUMA SCALE FOR ALCOHOL ABUSE

Since your eighteenth birthday:
1. Have you had any fractures or dislocations of bones or joints?
2. Have you been injured in an automobile accident?
3. Have you injured your head?
4. Have you been injured in an assault or fight? (Excluding sports.)
5. Have you been injured after drinking?

One point for each positive response. A score of 2 or more suggests alcohol abuse.

SOURCE: Reproduced with permission, from Skinner HA, Holt S, Schuller R, et al. Identification of alcohol abuse using laboratory tests and a history of trauma. *Ann Intern Med* 1984; 101:847–851.

gency room setting.[7] This set of questions is based on the fact that alcoholic patients are susceptible to frequent episodes of trauma.

In summary, several questionnaires are available to assist in identifying depression, alcohol abuse, and other psychiatric disorders. Some of these instruments can be self-administered. Any of them can be incorporated quite reasonably into a comprehensive medical interview. They yield quantitative data (scores) that can be compared with general guidelines or standards, but they usually do not in themselves yield a definitive diagnosis of the condition in question. Such questionnaires should be used to enhance your ability to assess the patient (case finding) for certain conditions that are often difficult to detect.

Patient Monitoring by Questionnaire

We should include one other useful function of questionnaires in the medical interview: monitoring of symptoms. It is often useful to have some quantitative or semiquantitative method of determining how much a patient's symptoms change over time. While traditionally we rely on patients' qualitative reports, certain chronic illnesses change slowly or cyclically, so even patients themselves may not be able to assess accurately the difference in their symptom patterns between one point and another point several weeks or months later. Various types of chronic infammatory arthritis, multiple sclerosis, and depression and other mental disorders are examples of such conditions. If symptom checklists or questionnaires are available, the cumulative symptom score on one occasion may be compared with scores obtained on other occasions. This method of symptom monitoring is frequently used in clinical depression—for example, where BDI or SDS scores obtained at successive visits may be used in helping to determine the effect of treatment.

COMPUTER-ASSISTED HISTORY TAKING

Many related applications use computers to improve the collection and interpretation of patient history data:

- Computers can be used to process and store information collected from questionnaires completed by patients before the clinical encounter, or by physicians during the encounter.

- Computers might be used interactively by a patient or by a health-care-team intermediary as a supplement to or replacement for a face-to-face interview. In such cases, from the clinician's point of view, the interactive program may yield a printout that enhances clinical efficiency. From the patient's point of view, interacting with a computer may provide a less-threatening setting than a face-to-face encounter with a physician for eliciting potentially embarrassing information.

- One might use computers diagnostically; in more sophisticated applications, computer programs can generate diagnostic possibilities and then implicitly (or in some cases explicitly) prompt physicians to seek further history and physical data from the patient to investigate these possibilities.

- In addition to obtaining information from the patient, computer programs might provide educational information or lifestyle modification instructions to the patient.

- Computers might be used as aids in teaching interviewing skills.

Acquisition of Patient Data

Computers have been employed, with varying degrees of sophistication, to assist the physician in acquiring patient data. Many physicians ask new patients to complete a general health survey before coming in for the initial examination; these data may then be entered into a computerized database by clerical assistants or by electronic means such as an optical scanner. Indeed, this use of computers was the earliest attempt at mechanizing the process of history taking and, though not sophisticated, is still a useful technique. In addition to providing a database of patient information, programs that use this technique can generate printed summaries that prepare the physician for a patient encounter, allowing the physician to focus more efficiently on the patient's complaints. Such questionnaires, however, are often time-consuming for the patient to complete and may be time-consuming to enter into the computer if an electronic scanner is not used. Additionally, this technique fails to take advantage of the interactive power of the computer.

Interactive computer-assisted history programs, in which the patient directly enters information, can use patient time and energy more efficiently through the use of branching algorithms. With such a technique, if a patient answers "no" to a general question, the program will bypass the related, more specific questions, much as you might do in a face-to-face interview. Thus, pertinent areas can be explored in some detail without annoying the user with a long list of irrelevant questions. Such an algorithm could also be used to give a patient pertinent lifestyle modification suggestions without subjecting him or her to superfluous information.

Other programs take advantage of stored medical knowledge to obtain information in a more intelligent manner. This field of investigation and application is rapidly changing. Earlier programs were limited to specific categories of disease (e.g., renal, pulmonary) or to stored information regarding the answers to a relatively small number of questions, but newer programs have wide applicability and enormous databases. The advent of CD-ROM technology has been particularly helpful in allowing the creation and general availability of such programs.

Advantages

There are several advantages to using computer-assisted history collection. Patients usually find the technique acceptable, and some reports indicate that the practice may result in the recording of more complete information. By collecting some data ahead of time, the physician might be able to focus more efficiently on selected areas during the actual interview. Additionally, patients may be more willing to disclose information on sensitive topics to a computer than to a physician. As an additional benefit, interactive computer sessions may be used to provide educational information.

Problems

Useful as the technique may be, computer-assisted history taking suffers from limitations that make it unlikely ever to replace the clinician-patient interview. Patients' responses to a computerized questionnaire are limited to yes/no or, at best, to categorical answers. The tendency to ask closed-ended questions may be exacerbated when the history is obtained by an intermediary using the computer for assistance. Use of such closed-ended questions may inhibit exploration of areas not specifically included in the questionnaire. Also, it is not unusual for the use of computers to increase (rather than decrease) the amount of time spent obtaining the history. Perhaps most importantly, clinicians know that important information is obtained not only from the patient responses per se, but also from the manner in which the patient replies and from subtle, nonverbal cues that can never be captured by a computer-assisted questionnaire.

Interactive computer programs also suffer one limitation that simpler, paper-and-pencil questionnaires do not. The programs demand that the patient complete the questionnaire at a computer in the physician's office. This, in turn, requires the physician to have available suitable computers that are dedicated almost exclusively to this purpose and located in a reasonably private area to ensure patient confidentiality. The use of computers also necessitates some sophistication on the part of the patient and may require that office personnel provide instruction. Now that the prices of microcomputers have fallen dramatically and many programs are "user- friendly," the option of having dedicated computers for interactive history taking is becoming increasingly attractive. Nonetheless, computer-obtained histories are best viewed as an adjunct to, rather than as a substitute for, traditionally obtained histories.

Computer-Assisted Medical Diagnosis

The types of programs just discussed are designed to accept historical input and then organize it as an aid to the physician's history taking. Systems are now available that can go several steps beyond this: they are designed to accept history, physical, and laboratory input and then suggest plausible diagnoses. A full discussion of medical expert systems and computer-assisted medical diagnosis is beyond the scope of this chapter; several good general reviews are included in the list of Suggested Readings.

S U M M A R Y : Questionnaires and Computers

Certain aspects of the medical interview that rely on focused questioning may be adapted to a questionnaire format. Patients may complete such questionnaires before a clinical encounter, or clinicians may use them to structure part of the medical interview. They are most useful:

- As reminders to ask for, or follow up on, certain information
- As case finding instruments, especially for psychiatric disorders
- As semiquantitative methods of monitoring patient symptoms

Interactive computer programs may also be used as adjuncts to history taking. In this rapidly developing field, interactive programs have many advantages over paper questionnaires, but they also have disadvantages—particularly, limited adaptability to the clinical setting. Computer programs are potentially helpful in medical diagnosis and patient education. Regardless of their level of sophistication, these programs are not likely to replace the health-care professional as primary data gatherer, diagnostician, and teacher.

References

1. Zimmerman M, Coryell W. The validity of a self-report questionnaire for diagnosing major depressive disorder. *Arch Gen Psychiatry* 1988; 45:738–740.
2. Zung WK. A self-rating depression scale. *Arch Gen Psychiatry* 1965; 12:63–70.
3. Seltzer ML. The Michigan Alcoholism Screening Test: The quest for a new diagnostic instrument. *Am J Psychiatry* 1971; 127:1653–1658.
4. Spitzer RL, William JB, Kroenke K, et al.: Utility of a new procedure of diagnosing mental disorders in primary care: The PRIME-MD 1000 study. *JAMA* 1994; 272:1749–1756.
5. Coulehan JL, Schulberg HC, Block MR. The efficiency of depression questionnaires for case finding in primary medical care. *J Gen Intern Med* 1989; 4:461–467.
6. Cyr MG, Wartman SA. The effectiveness of routine screening questions in the detection of alcoholism. *JAMA* 1988; 259:51–54.
7. Skinner HA, Holt S, Schuller R, et al. Identification of alcohol abuse using laboratory tests and a history of trauma. *Ann Intern Med* 1984; 101:847–851.

Suggested Readings

De Vore PA. Computerized geriatric assessment for geriatric care management. *Aging* 1995; 7:194–196.

Forsstrom JJ, Dalton KJ. Artificial neural networks for decision support in clinical medicine. *Ann Med* 1995; 27:509–517.

Johnson KB, Feldman MJ. Medical informatics and pediatrics. Decision-support systems. *Arch Pediatr Adolesc Med* 1995; 149:1371–1380.

Miller RA. Medical diagnostic decision support systems—past, present, and future: A threaded bibliography and brief commentary. *J Am Med Inform Assoc* 1994; 1:8–27.

CHAPTER 13

Is This Case Serious or Not?

• • •

CLINICAL JUDGMENT IN THE MEDICAL INTERVIEW

. . . To Ivan Ilych only one question was important: was his case serious or not? But the doctor ignored that inappropriate question. From his point of view it was not the one under consideration, the real question was to decide between a floating kidney, chronic catarrh or appendicitis. It was not a question of life or death, but one between a floating kidney and appendicitis.

Leo Tolstoy, *The Death of Ivan Ilych*

Throughout this text we maintain that most of the information you need to make appropriate diagnoses and to take care of your patients comes from the clinical encounter. Although we emphasize a thorough and holistic approach to the patient, uncertainty and ambiguity are inevitable in patient care. Clinicians rarely have access to all relevant data; diagnostic and therapeutic decisions are almost always made in the context of uncertainty. We use various devices to minimize uncertainty, but in the long run, usually we act with incomplete data. For example, based on past experience and epidemiologic knowledge, we assume that a 30-year-old man without gastrointestinal symptoms does not require a sigmoidoscopy as part of his evaluation. Can we say with 100 percent certainty that he has no colonic polyps? No, we cannot, but the probability is very, very low. A good history is the most effective and efficient way to ensure that our "negative" assumption is correct. If the patient tells us he had an episode of rectal bleeding or has a family history of intestinal polyposis, the probabilities change and a sigmoidoscopy may well be indicated.

All diagnostic and therapeutic decisions are, in a sense, experiments.[1] We formulate a hypothesis, manipulate variables, and see what happens. Although we weigh probabilities, risks, benefits, experience, knowledge, and expert opinions, in the long run we are still left with hypotheses—some very well supported, some questionable—that have to be tested. Are these symptoms really caused by this particular disease? Is this finding important? Will this medication actually help the patient? Learning to accept and work within uncertainty is a major part of your professional education. Sound clinical judgment is the logical and empathic approach to decision making within this uncertain environment.

Figure 13–1 illustrates the feedback loop of clinical judgment as it occurs during a medical interview. Elements of process or technique allow the interviewer to obtain certain data (content), which ultimately must be organized into the traditional sections of a medical history. Even in the earliest phases of the interview, however, the clinician formulates hypotheses that influence the continuing process of data collection. Figure 13–1 indicates four different types of clinical hypotheses.[1] A central concern of clinical practice is differential diagnosis, or formulating hypotheses about the patient's disease process. However, the accuracy of differential diagnosis depends partly on a set of preliminary hypotheses about the quality of the story itself: How does it fit together? Did X happen before or after Y? Is the narrative plausible? The clinician also generates hypotheses about the patient's personality and interactive style: What sort of coping style does he or she have? What might one expect in terms of adherence to treatment recommendations or behavioral change? Finally, when problems arise in the interview, one must also consider hypotheses about the clinical encounter itself: What is going wrong here? Why do I feel so frustrated or uncomfortable? Why is the patient so angry? In Chapter 10 we considered various hypotheses about interviewing problems that arise when caring for so-called difficult patients.

We consider in this chapter some topics raised by the uncertainty that is an everyday part of clinician-patient interactions. First, we discuss probability and utility as components of clinical judgment. Next, we present a list of decision-making guidelines that help inform clinical judgment. Finally, we review a variety of common psychologic biases that have the potential to distort our decision making in the interview.

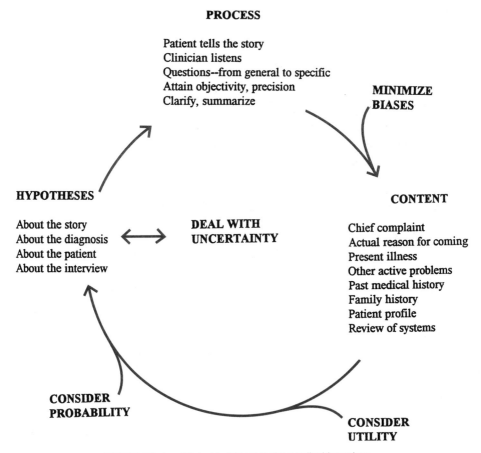

FIGURE 13–1. Clinical judgment in the medical interview.

COMPONENTS OF CLINICAL JUDGMENT

When you first learn to interview and examine patients, one of your main goals is to be complete. You imagine that the "big picture" will somehow click into place, if only you collect all of the available data. Some of your preceptors may emphasize completeness as if there were a certain finite body of medical facts that, once obtained, would magically fit together like a jigsaw puzzle, allowing you to generate diagnoses and therapeutic plans more or less mechanistically. Students who enter the clinical setting accustomed to textbook learning are particularly susceptible to thinking that "reading" patients is a straightforward process of getting through as many "pages of text" as possible, with little judgment along the way. Later, as you think carefully about what you "read," its meaning will cohere.

If you collect data in this fashion during clinical encounters, you will exhaust both yourself and the patient. In reality, as they proceed through the encounter, clinicians constantly generate guesses or hypotheses about what might be wrong with the patient and what could be done to help, and they direct the interview (and subsequent diagnostic strategy) to provide data to evaluate these hypotheses and possibly generate new ones.[2] This iterative process, which is called the **hypothetico-deductive method**, is quite different from the inductive method, in which the collection of a huge amount of data might allow one to generate a diagnostic conclusion.

Clinical Probability

Investigators have shown that experienced physicians generate a variety of hypotheses about what causes the patient's problem within the first 2 minutes, and often within the first 30 seconds, of beginning the clinical encounter.[2] Data gathering constantly changes its character based on what has gone before. Clinicians have a fairly limited ability to juggle hypotheses that might explain a given problem; usually no more than five hypotheses are considered at any time.[2] They then design their questioning and other testing to obtain data that either enhance or decrease the **probability** of one or more of the hypotheses. They continue this process until one hypothesis stands out sufficiently from the others that it can be acted upon. Thus, the clinical method, just like the scientific method, does not involve first gathering an enormous amount of data and then later seeing how all the parts fit together; rather, most of the data are collected for the purpose of testing hypotheses. For example, on the most elementary level, as soon as you walk into the room and see that the patient is a woman of a particular age, you know that some diagnoses are possible, whereas others are impossible.

The nature of this process means that probability plays a major role in clinical judgment during the interview. We ask questions that are most likely to clarify the problem and we use the treatment that is most likely to help. Ideally, probability testing requires:

- A broad knowledge of pathophysiology and therapeutics
- Prior probability (or prevalence) estimates for the given disease, based on textbook facts and, later, on our own experience
- A logical approach for estimating changes in the probability

Good clinicians integrate these functions in making clinical judgments all the time but frequently find it difficult to differentiate the elements of this process so that they can be stated explicitly.

Clinical Utility

Clinical judgment is conditioned by the concept known as **utility,** as well as by probability. Diagnoses or decisions are not ends in themselves but rather tools for making the patient feel better. Thus, we want to pay particular attention to certain kinds of diagnostic hypotheses even when they do not seem to be the most probable explanation or even very likely. For example, the **seriousness** of diseases must be considered. Serious diseases must be ruled out much more aggressively than mild or self-limited diseases. Even though a random positive test result for occult blood in the stool of a healthy, asymptomatic individual most likely does not indicate cancer, it is medically appropriate to do a thorough evaluation of the lower GI tract in someone with such an unexplained finding. It would be poor judgment to ignore the results of that test (i.e., the stool guaiac), even though the risk of cancer in a person with a single positive test result may be less than 5 percent.

Treatability is another aspect of utility. There is no point in pursuing diagnosis for the sake of diagnosis unless it can have some benefit for the patient. Simply learning the diagnosis and satisfying our own curiosity about the factors that led to the outcome may, in fact, have no value for the patient. Our decisions should be dictated by utility for the patient, not utility for us, unless the patient has voluntarily enrolled in an experimental protocol. There is no sense in doing a liver biopsy on an alcoholic patient who comes to the hospital with abnormal liver function tests once we have ascertained that the test result will have nothing to do with the patient's subsequent management. If in the future the same patient has recurrent episodes of abdominal problems or abnormal liver function, we might question the hypothesis that his problem is alcoholic liver disease, and perhaps a biopsy would then be indicated. But even then the decision must be dictated by what is best for the patient. Our desire to know is not necessarily best for the patient, especially when the risks and costs of further tests are high, as is the case with complex, invasive studies.

The patient's own assessment of usefulness is of paramount value, although health-care professionals often have a major impact on the patient's beliefs about utility. We do not believe, as some ethical and legal commentators suggest, that all medical decisions can or should always be made entirely independently by the rational patient. In fact, sick people tend to trust their physicians and often do not want to be burdened with multiple decisions, even when they fully understand the general nature and consequences of the options.[3] Investigators have found that informed consent, although espoused by most patients, is not so highly valued by them when faced with actual decisions about their own medical care. Rather than thinking through all the alternatives, patients tend to rely on their doctors' advice, expecting fidelity and advocacy in their relationship.[4] Fidelity, however, depends on the clinician's understanding of the patient. An interviewer who helps a patient express his or her values and allows the patient to ask questions will learn what facts, from an array of many, this particular patient needs to know to make a decision. The patient's value system and decisions about whether to accept medical care influence questions of negotiation and education, as considered in Chapters 14 and 15.

JUDGMENT GUIDELINES FOR THE MEDICAL INTERVIEW

These concepts of probability and utility, combined with knowledge of basic interviewing skills, serve as the basis for a set of **guidelines** for improving your clinical judgment during the interview. The list of guidelines in Table 13–1 summarizes thinking skills that contribute to effective clinical judg-

TABLE 13–1   GUIDELINES FOR IMPROVING CLINICAL JUDGMENT

Guidelines for Generating Hypotheses

- **Probability:** Consider the most common diagnoses first.
- **Utility:** Consider diagnoses more seriously if effective therapy is available, if treatment would be significantly different than that of competing diagnoses, or if failure to treat would hurt the patient.
- **Narrative thread:** Consider diagnoses more seriously if they are consistent with the patient's whole story, not just one part of it.
- **Interpersonal thread:** Consider diagnoses more seriously if they are consistent with all the data, including data about the person.
- **Multiple, competing hypotheses**: Avoid making "snap" diagnoses. Think of a number of diagnostic possibilities compatible with the chief complaint and data obtained in the early part of the medical interview.

Guidelines for Testing Hypotheses

- **Screen and branch:** Develop screening tactics to avoid unnecessarily detailed examinations. Develop branching procedures.
- **Plan:** Form a reasoned plan to test your hypotheses. There should be a reason for every piece of data you plan to gather.
- **Harm versus benefit**: Consider the harm, benefit, and cost of each test you order.
- **Clinical utility:** Never order tests whose results will not logically make a difference in the decision-making process.

Guidelines for Evaluating Hypotheses

- **Revision:** Continually revise probabilities as you collect more data; then alter your plan accordingly.
- **Disconfirmatory evidence**: Seek evidence that tends to rule out a diagnostic alternative, as well as evidence that tends to confirm it.
- **Multiple problems:** Consider the possibility that a patient with multiple symptoms or complaints may well have more than one disease.

ment during the medical interview and physical examination; the same skills serve as the basis for developing further strategies for diagnosis and management.[2]

BIAS IN CLINICAL JUDGMENT

We are all subject to certain psychological **biases** (Table 13–2) that can distort our clinical thinking.[5] In the interview these biases distort our hearing and understanding of the patient's symptoms and change the strategy of our hypothetico-deductive approach. These biases might make a particular diagnosis feel more probable or less probable than it really is; or make a particular strategy seem more useful or less useful than the facts would warrant. As human beings, we are all subject to errors in judgment, but we can minimize these errors by bringing them into the open and understanding just what they are and how they occur.

Availability

The bias of **availability** means that the clinician's assessment of how probable a diagnosis is relates to how easy it is for instances or occurrences of that disease to be brought to mind. This is simply another way of saying that the things that you are more familiar with or knowledgeable about appear to be more likely than uncertain or obscure items. A diagnosis might seem more probable than it really is if, for example, you have seen a patient who proved to have a similar diagnosis last week or you have just been reading about a certain disease in your textbook. Within the interview, you might go to a series of closed-ended or leading questions to discover what you suspect, thereby shutting out other symptoms that point to the real problem. For example, if you have just read the chapter on lymphomas, you may think that your patient with the chief complaint of "swollen glands" has Hodgkin's disease until proven otherwise. You might ask first about night sweats and weight loss, only later finding out that his 10-year-old son had a similar illness last week and that other symptoms suggest the much more likely simple streptococcal infection.

TABLE 13–2   PSYCHOLOGIC BIASES IN ESTIMATING PROBABILITY AND UTILITY

Availability	Anchoring and adjustment
Representativeness	Rule-in favoritism
Sunk costs	Occam's razor
Completeness	

Such bias often leads to a failure within the interview to obtain data needed to make the correct diagnosis. Here is an interview of a 38-year-old patient with abdominal pain. The interviewer has been reading about peptic ulcer disease:

Dr: Tell me what brought you to the clinic today.
Pt: Well, my stomach has been acting up for the past few weeks.
Dr: Does food make it better or worse?
Pt: That's hard to say, it depends on what I eat.
Dr: How about antacids?
Pt: Antacids?
Dr: Things like Maalox or Tagamet. Have you tried anything like that?
Pt: I think that might help. It helps the gas sometimes.

Notice the poor interviewing technique here. The interviewer fails to obtain information about the location of the pain (which happened to be lower abdominal, not epigastric). Instead, the interviewer jumps into a series of closed-ended questions intended to support a diagnosis of peptic ulcer disease. Notice the patient's attempt to please the interviewer with the "correct" response ("I think that might help"). In reality, this patient suffered from lactose intolerance causing lower abdominal pain, gaseousness, and diarrhea.

In a similar way, a subspecialist is likely to see diseases in his or her subspecialty as occurring more frequently than they really do in the general population or among people with the same set of symptoms who go to primary care doctors. Gastroenterologists are more likely than other physicians to diagnose GI disease, not only because their patients tend, of course, to have clear-cut GI symptom-complexes but also because gastroenterologists overvalue GI diagnoses among patients who have symptom-complexes that are also compatible with non-GI diagnoses.

Representativeness

Representativeness is another frequent psychologic bias, particularly among physicians who stick closely to their textbooks and clinical literature. These clinicians often think a rare disease is very probable if a patient has the representative or classic symptoms of that disease. Let us say a disease has five characteristic symptoms but is extremely rare, occurring in only one out of every million people. The five symptoms might be dizziness, right upper quadrant abdominal pain, frequent headaches, difficulty sleeping, and waking up in the morning with muscle stiffness. Unfortunately, each of these symptoms is also quite common by itself. Although a patient who has all five at once is more likely to have the rare disease, ordinary or more prevalent diseases are still the most probable explanation for the illness. Even though the patient provides a representative picture, common diseases are more likely to explain his or her problem than a rare disease. This does not mean that correct clinical judgment would never allow for making a rare diagnosis, but it does mean that pursuing such a diagnosis usually has more to do with utility than with probability. Early in a clinician's medical career, when he or she has had little practical experience with the prevalence of diseases, every disease seems as likely as any other, and every symptom seems as likely to represent a rare disease as a common one.

Sunk Costs

If a certain amount of money or effort has already been invested in pursuing a given diagnostic strategy, the outcome or yield from that strategy may appear more likely than it really is, and the physician may continue further tests so as not to "waste" those tests already performed. This is the bias called **sunk costs.** Let us say that a patient is ill with general muscle aches, malaise, and intermittent fevers. He also had some nonspecific abdominal pain which, when you first take the history, you believe suggests a GI abnormality. You then order an upper GI x-ray series (normal), and on subsequent discussion with the patient you find that the GI symptoms are really not as important a part of the syndrome as you first thought. The bias of sunk costs tends to make you feel more compelled to complete the GI work-up (with a barium enema and flexible sigmoidoscopy, for example), rather than to leave the GI symptoms "hanging."

In a very broad sense, the fact that you have a hypothesis, or several of them, tends to make you look more carefully at observations relevant to those hypotheses and to ignore or minimize other observations. You must have a frame of reference for your thinking. Clear thinking necessarily leads more and more strongly in a given direction, simply because the remaining hypotheses are judged very probable, very useful, or both. The bias of sunk costs is an exaggeration of this process, which leads to focusing too intently on a diagnosis simply because you are invested in it. Then you may not be receptive to the implications of new data that should change the way you think about the problem.

Completeness

One way to categorize mistakes in medicine is to divide them into errors of commission and errors of omission. You may err by doing the wrong thing or failing to do the right one. In evaluating patients, we often talk of doing a medical test "for completeness' sake." This pat phrase makes it sound like **completeness** is a powerful entity that demands our service, independent of the needs of the patient. In fact, if we make clinical decisions for completeness' sake, these decisions may result in consequences that are harmful to the patient.

All this is another way of saying that errors of commission are generally more sanctioned in medicine than errors of omission. You rarely get into trouble with your peers if you order extra studies or make the examination more complete than necessary, unless you order a very invasive and expensive test that is obviously unnecessary. On the other hand, you are frequently asked to justify yourself if you do not order a diagnostic test that may be only mildly relevant to a particular illness, or that is relevant but unnecessary because its result will not change a therapeutic decision. We make decisions about completeness all the time when we interview patients. We may decide, for example, to forgo the history of childhood diseases in an 85-year-old woman with hypertension, or to skip the sexual history in a new patient who presents with acute back pain. We often feel, however, that omitting certain parts of the history is less acceptable than taking a too-invasive history. We continually weigh the value of the information likely to be obtained against the limits of the patient's tolerance to be interviewed because he or she is too sick or too tired or would feel that certain matters are too private.

Many physicians justify completeness by a call to "defensive medicine." They claim that they have to do a CT scan in a young man who has a bump on his head and who never lost consciousness because the case may end up in court some day. The issue of malpractice liability was discussed briefly in Chapter 9. Let us reiterate here that negligence claims usually stem from poor communication and patient dissatisfaction because of poor rapport, misunderstandings, physician inaccessibility, and personality clashes. Good interviewing skills help avoid or minimize all of these.

The bias of completeness is closely related to the bias of sunk costs. If you order enough tests for the sake of completeness, occasionally one of them will be truly useful. But how many errors of commission, with all their attendant costs and risks, will you have to make in order to prevent one error of omission?

Anchoring and Adjustment

Availability, representativeness, sunk costs, and completeness can be observed every day in the practice of medicine. The bias called **anchoring and adjustment** is a little more arcane. Physicians use some rough estimate of subjective probability to start with and then anchor their opinions at that level, using an adjustment factor to revise opinions upward or downward as a result of new information. It is psychologically difficult to condense vast ranges of probability into the diagnostic problem frame, particularly when you know the patient is ill and there is a 100 percent probability that something is wrong. What can you do with a differential diagnosis in which one hypothesis has a 75 percent probability and another a 0.001 percent probability? Physicians cope with this problem by anchoring their estimates in a middle range, so that very unlikely diagnoses get overvalued and likely diagnoses often get undervalued. The adjustment factor after considering new evidence tends to be smaller in either direction than is really warranted by the facts. The net effect is that judgments hover toward the middle level of probability, and clinicians often consider diseases that have vastly different likelihood with only moderately different degrees of seriousness while pursuing their diagnostic strategy.

Rule-in Favoritism

Because medicine demands action, there is also a bias in favor of making the diagnosis out of the array of hypotheses available. Clinicians often seek out and evaluate evidence to support their main hypotheses but are less aggressive in seeking out evidence that could rule out this hypothesis. This tendency might be called **rule-in favoritism**. Within the interview, for example, you might actively seek symptoms such as nausea, radiation to the jaw or left arm, and sweating to support your hypothesis that the patient's chest pain is due to coronary insufficiency. You may choose not to ask if the pain occurs upon lying down or is relieved by antacids (to try to rule out esophageal reflux). The worth of an open-ended question such as "Did you notice anything else?" is its power to elicit data we simply forgot or did not think of because of this bias.

Occam's Razor

We should also mention the tendency to try to make one diagnosis, rather than several. This principle of parsimony is a reasonable clinical guideline, a heuristic that all students of medicine should consider when evaluating the patient's history and physical findings. It is called **Occam's razor**, named after William of Occam, a 14th-century scholastic philosopher. In medicine this principle means that we should try to explain the entire illness—all the symptoms—with one diagnosis. While this is a good "rule of thumb" to keep in mind, it is certainly not always correct, especially in these days of multiple chronic and degenerative diseases. In particular, the concurrence of two common diseases (e.g., diabetes mellitus and peptic ulcer) is a more likely explanation of the symptom-complex of abdominal pain, vomiting, polyuria, and polydipsia than is the occurrence of one rare disease (e.g., acute intermittent porphyria). Occam's razor supports the bias of representativeness when it makes us favor latching onto an uncommon diagnosis to avoid considering the less intellectually satisfying alternative of partitioning the diagnosis of the illness among several more probable explanations.

S U M M A R Y : Clinical Judgment in the Interview

Good clinical judgment is the logical and empathic approach to decision making in a context of uncertainty. In this chapter we have delineated aspects of clinical decision making that relate to the process and content of the medical interview. Clinical judgment (or in the medical history, differential diagnosis) requires assessments of probability and utility for each hypothesis as you interview the patient. To estimate utility, consider the seriousness and treatability of the disease in question, as well as the patient's own goals and values. Guidelines allow the clinician to put these abstract concepts of decision making into practice when taking a patient's medical history (p. 243).

Certain psychologic biases tend to distort assessments of probability or utility in the interview and, thereby, impair clinical decision making. These include the biases of:

- Availability
- Representativeness
- Sunk costs
- Completeness
- Anchoring and adjustment
- Rule-in favoritism
- Occam's razor

Each bias may adversely impact clinical judgment unless the clinician minimizes its influence during the diagnostic interview.

References

1. Platt FW, McMath JC. Clinical hypocompetence: The interview. *Ann Intern Med* 1979; 91:898–902.
2. Elstein AS, Schulman LS, Sprafka SA. *Medical Problem Solving: An Analysis of Clinical Reasoning.* Cambridge, MA, Harvard University Press, 1978.
3. Mazur DJ. Why the goals of informed consent are not realized: Treatise on informed consent for the primary care physician. *J Gen Intern Med* 1988; 3:370–380.
4. Brody H. Transparency: Informed consent in primary care. *Hastings Center Rep* 1989; Sept/Oct:5–9.
5. Tversky A, Kahneman D. Judgment under uncertainty: Heuristics and biases. *Science* 1974; 185: 1124–1131.

Suggested Readings

Feinstein AR. An analysis of diagnostic reasoning. II: The strategy of intermediate decisions. *Yale J Biol Med* 1973; 46:264–283.

Feinstein AR. "Clinical judgment" revisited: The distraction of quantitative models. *Ann Intern Med* 1994; 120:799–805.

Lilford RJ, Thornton JD. Decision logic in medical practice. *J R Coll Physicians (Lond)* 1992; 26:400–412.

CHAPTER 14

For the Moment at Least I Actually Became Them

• • •

UNDERSTANDING THE PATIENT'S BELIEFS AND VALUES

. . . for the moment at least I actually became them; whoever they should be, so that when I detached myself from them at the end of a half-hour of intense concentration over some illness which was affecting them, it was as though I was awakening from a sleep.

William Carlos Williams, *The Autobiography*

In this chapter we discuss the central importance in the medical interview of understanding the patient's values and beliefs regarding health and illness and expectations regarding therapy. By "values" we mean the patient's fundamental moral and existential commitments and, in particular, how those commitments are manifest in the patient's attitudes and behavior. By "beliefs" we mean both general and specific understandings about what causes

251

illness, how it develops, what you can do about it, and what will happen if you don't do anything. Values and beliefs determine expectations. The first two sections of the chapter deal briefly with the ways that values and beliefs affect patients' decision making and behavior regarding illness. The next section indicates a number of clinical situations in which explicit questioning about health beliefs is likely to contribute to accurate diagnosis and effective treatment. Finally, we present a framework for inquiring about the patient's interpretation of his or her illness.

THE PATIENT'S VALUES AND YOUR OWN

Values lie at the core of any clinician-patient encounter. The ill person values life and health, as does the clinician. Presumably, the patient also values the clinician's help, and the clinician respects (values) the patient. In many cases these implicit commitments are sufficient. However, the dramatic growth in our ability to treat chronic and degenerative disease has brought the need to explore values more explicitly. This is most obviously true in the care of dying patients. One person may value the sanctity of life at all costs, whereas another places greater value on quality of life. Such commitments and the health-care decisions that derive from them are embodied in advance directives (see p. 222). Similarly, in the care of the chronically ill, you will find that some patients place a very high premium on personal independence and self-determination, but others are more oriented toward family relationships and interdependence. Culture and religion make substantial contributions to the development and maintenance of human values. In some cases, specific religious values have a significant impact on medical treatment. For example, if a patient highly values the "sanctity of life," that will affect his or her decisions about withholding or withdrawing life-sustaining therapy. Similarly, "spiritual purity" influences Jehovah's Witnesses in deciding not to accept blood transfusions. In other cases, cultural values play a major role in decision making; among Native Americans, for example, families engage in a group decision-making process that appears to conflict with the usual American ideal of individual autonomy.

In interviewing seriously or chronically ill patients, the clinician should also be aware of his or her own underlying values. Health-care professionals tend to assume that medical explanations for illness phenomena and medically indicated forms of treatment represent "reality" rather than beliefs, and are self-evident. This reflects the high value we place on attempting to control the world (and our lives) through the use of medical science and our tendency to undervalue ambiguity and "unscientific" explanations. Some clinicians have more tolerance than others for patients with alternate values. One of the first steps toward respecting and trying to understand patients who disagree with us (respect and empathy, see Chap. 2) is a commitment to self-awareness.

UNDERSTANDING WHAT THE PATIENT BELIEVES

The human experience of illness is never value-free or meaning-free. From the time people first become ill, unless they're unconscious, they try to figure out what's wrong with them and why it happened. Nonetheless, clinicians tend to view their patients as **empty vessels** and to see their own job as pouring the vessel full of medical information about diagnosis and treatment. A common view is that good clinical practice includes "educating" patients in this way. Sometimes clinicians patiently explain disease processes again and again on repeated visits to no avail; patients just don't seem to understand. They don't take their medications properly; they seem to have little or no concern about their health. In such cases, clinicians tend to throw up their hands in frustration: "That woman's completely noncompliant. There's nothing I can do." "I've told him time and again, but he's just so thick-headed and self-destructive."

In fact, the empty-vessel metaphor is based on an incorrect premise; the cup is already full of information, beliefs, and values. The cup is full of a solution that constitutes much of the patient's personal identity and determines his or her experience of illness and expectations of the clinician. Thus, in cases of significant illness, the clinician needs to identify and understand these pre-existing beliefs and values before he or she can add an appropriate "dose" of medical information and facilitate the creation of a new, therapeutic solution.

It is useful to think of health beliefs as lying at various points along two related axes (Fig. 14–1). One is the continuum from cultural belief systems to personal and very idiosyncratic beliefs. The other axis ranges from coherent, integrated beliefs that are important aspects of personal identity to isolated or fragmented bits of information ("info-fragments") that the person picks up and may just as easily discard. Integrated belief systems are embedded in deeply held values.

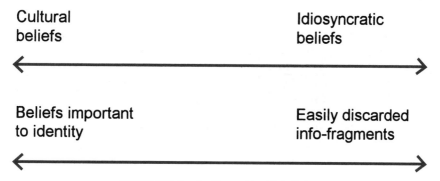

FIGURE 14–1. Continua of health beliefs.

Cultural Belief Systems

It is perhaps easiest for clinicians to understand the importance of health beliefs in cross-cultural settings, in which patients clearly have a different ethnic or cultural background from that of the health-care professional. In our multicultural society, it is now quite common for Anglo clinicians to encounter Hispanic patients, for Indian clinicians to work with Vietnamese patients, for Russian clinicians to see Haitian patients, and vice versa. Language is the most obvious barrier to communication (see p. 39). Even when the patient or clinician has learned the other's language, it may be difficult to express deeply held beliefs or complex medical explanations in a second tongue.

The fact that a person appears as a patient in a medical office does not necessarily imply that he or she shares the Western, scientific belief system regarding the etiology and treatment of illness. For example, non-Hispanic physicians who treat Hispanic patients may encounter problems by inadvertently prescribing a "hot" medicine for a "hot" disease. Many Puerto Ricans, Dominicans, and Mexican-Americans subscribe to a traditional folk physiology that requires a balance between "hot" and "cold" humors for health; illness occurs when there is an imbalance. In this culture certain diseases are characterized as cold and others as hot; medicines and other treatments are also divided in this way. To restore the appropriate balance, a cold illness must be treated with a hot medicine, and vice versa. The unsuspecting physician who prescribes hot for hot may well have a reluctant and noncompliant patient.[1] Similar notions of illness as imbalance or dysharmony occur in Chinese (yin/yang) and Native American cultures. In each case, prescribed medical treatment may either be consistent or inconsistent with culturally recommended therapy. The Western clinician must be able to understand enough of the patient's belief system to be able to recommend a treatment plan that is synergistic with those beliefs.

Culture differences may also lead clinicians and patients to interpret illness **language** differently. A striking example (not so prevalent as it once was) is the "high blood-low blood" folk physiology in black and rural white populations in the south.[2] In these cultures, people confuse hypertension (high blood pressure) with "high blood," which they interpret as excessive blood volume. This condition is believed to cause strokes because excess blood tends to back up into the brain. The same people use the term "low blood" for anemia, which, they believe, puts a strain on the person's heart. Thus, high blood and low blood are considered opposites when, in fact, the two diseases involve completely different organ systems. It is difficult, then, for patients with these beliefs to accept the notion that they can be hypertensive and anemic at the same time.

Personal Beliefs

The use of cross-cultural examples to illustrate the importance of health beliefs may, however, have an unfortunate and unintended consequence. Like most people, clinicians tend to look upon "culture" as something that applies only to others (the more exotic the difference, the more this belief is held), not to themselves or to people who look and talk like themselves. Such clinicians may readily acknowledge that illness-related beliefs make a difference when treating people of other cultures, but they ignore the wide spectrum of folk physiology and healing practices presented by ordinary people in our society, regardless of age, cultural background, or education. This represents, in part, a **cultural blind spot**; that is, our own beliefs seem so obviously true that we don't realize they are culturally determined.

Although culture may provide the context, personal beliefs develop from a variety of sources: childhood experience, formal education, interactions with family and friends, television, newspapers, and so forth. One's conceptualization of illness, threshold for seeking professional help, and expectation for cure are all based on one's personal belief system. Most people have not studied medical textbooks, nor do they necessarily share the same blind faith in science that health-care professionals often have. When one is sick, it is difficult to believe that the illness is a random event, a matter of probability—for example, 22 percent of persons exposed to a certain virus become clinically ill and, of these, 14 percent develop jaundice. "Yes," you ask, "but why me? Why did I get sick now, rather than last week or last year? What does it mean?"

One type of personal meaning derives from the patient's underlying value system and personality[3] (Table 14–1). If a patient views her illness as a punishment (e.g., for putting her mother in a nursing home), she may believe that she needs to atone for the sin. This could compromise her ability to get well. Another patient who attributes his heart attack to personal weakness (e.g., "I just don't have what it takes") may well deny the seriousness of his medical problem and resist treatment. Another type of personal meaning has to do with concepts of how illness happens; for example, high blood pressure is caused by stress, a cold is caused by sitting in a draft, cancer is caused by high-energy power lines. Sometimes these meanings are derived from more extensive belief systems. Some patients, for instance, believe that good nutrition and vitamin supplements are "natural" methods of healing and are, therefore, more effective than medications. Others may think, "A lot of illness comes from spinal subluxations; when I'm sick I should visit my chiropractor." Often, however, beliefs about illness are fragmented and contradictory, falling into the category of simple misinformation.

TABLE 14–1   PERSONAL ORIENTATIONS TOWARD ILLNESS AND POSSIBLE RESPONSES

Personal Orientation	Responses
Illness as challenge	Adapt actively
	Generate rational, task-oriented behavior
Illness as punishment	Feel anxious, depressed, or angry
	Possibly see opportunity for atonement
Illness as enemy	Be ready to fight, flee, or surrender
	Blame others
	Feel hostility or aggressiveness
Illness as weakness	Feel shame or loss of control
	Conceal or deny illness
Illness as relief	Reduce other obligations
Illness as strategy	Use illness as strategic ploy to manipulate
	Adopt dependent role or clinging
Illness as loss or damage	Experience depression, hostility, or resistance
	Be prone to suicide
Illness as value	Take opportunity to reflect
	Expand personality
	Use illness as creative catalyst

SOURCE: Adapted from Lipowski ZJ. Physical illness, the individual and the coping process. *Psychiatry Med* 1970; 1:91–102.

MISINFORMATION

Nowadays, people are constantly exposed to health-related "info-fragments" from television, radio, magazines, and newspapers. From these a person may garner a variety of "facts" and opinions, many of which will be inconsistent with others. In today's diet-frenzied culture, for instance, a patient may learn in one article that, in order to be healthy, he or she should eat a low-fat diet; another article will stridently recommend a low-carbohydrate diet; a third will cite "scientific studies" that "prove" the efficacy of a low-protein diet. But how can your diet be low in all three major foodstuffs? This inconsistency may be obvious to someone who understands the biochemistry of nutrition, but to many patients the three beliefs about diet are not necessarily inconsistent. Yet the simultaneous presence of these three info-fragments makes it very difficult for the patient to eat reasonably and contributes to diet-anxiety. An enormous number of such info-fragments swirl through our popular culture:

- All men should frequently have a screening blood test for prostate cancer.
- All women should frequently be tested for osteoporosis.

- A lot of cancer is caused by electromagnetic radiation from power lines.
- Vitamin E supplements relieve impotence.
- Vitamin C cures the common cold.
- Chelation therapy helps get rid of atherosclerosis.
- Cancer can be cured by stimulating the immune system.

To many people, the world is awash with new and exciting medical "discoveries" every day.

Health-care professionals may contribute to this misinformation. Consider the following excerpt from a conversation between a physician and a patient seeking medical care because of epigastric pain and "heartburn."

Pt: I take shots for allergies and I take two aspirins every day for my blood pressure. . . . I don't eat any sugar, any salt.

Dr: Two aspirins for . . .

Pt: Every morning.

Dr: For what, why do you take that?

Pt: Trying, trying to thin out my blood to keep my pressure down, I try to keep it around 100.

Dr: I see.

Later in the same interview the patient comes back to the issue of aspirin and blood pressure in this way:

Pt: But I always take two aspirins, I've taken two aspirins for years.

Dr: Where did you get into that habit?

Pt: Ah, when I was in the military in '78 and '79.

Dr: Um humm.

Pt: A German doctor told me that, ah, if you take two aspirins with milk in the morning, he says, it lowers your blood pressure and thins things out.

Dr: Um humm.

Pt: And I've always . . . my blood pressure is always like 100, 110, it's real low.

If you accept this person's basic premise, he has a perfectly logical belief regarding aspirin and blood pressure. He assumes that high blood pressure is caused by "thick" blood. If so, and if aspirin thins the blood, it is reasonable to take aspirin to prevent hypertension. This particular belief is likely to be simply a piece of misinformation. (It is, however, somewhat similar to the cultural "high blood-low blood" beliefs described earlier.) The physician could easily remedy this misinformation by explaining that blood pressure and blood coagulation involve two entirely different physiologic systems. Such an explanation would be particularly important if, in fact, this patient has gastritis or peptic ulcer and should, therefore, no longer use aspirin, or if he subsequently develops hypertension and antihypertensive medications are recommended.

WHEN DO YOU NEED TO KNOW MORE ABOUT THE PATIENT'S BELIEFS?

Although all ill persons are likely to have interpreted their illnesses, it is inefficient and unnecessary always to ask about these beliefs as part of the medical history. Most patients have some faith in scientific medicine, or else they would not have appeared in your office or come to the hospital. If you are empathic and demonstrate your clinical competence, patients will develop faith in you personally, in addition to whatever faith they have in medical care. By simply doing a good job, you will help change their interpretation of their illness, if, in fact, that interpretation conflicts with "reality" or with appropriate medical treatment. However, there are certain situations in which belief factors play a more significant role, and you will not be able to optimize the diagnostic and therapeutic power of the encounter unless you understand and deal with them.

How can you tell if you are dealing with a situation in which belief factors may be significantly influencing the patient's illness behavior and response to therapy? One type of "red flag" is when a chronically ill patient appears always to be poorly controlled despite effective medications and close monitoring. You suspect that the patient is not taking the medication as prescribed, but you don't understand why and don't know what to do. Often, you become angry with such patients because they do not seem to understand simple English ("I told her time and again, and explained the pills over and over, but I can tell she doesn't take them") or appear to be unconcerned about their condition, or self-destructive ("What is he trying to do, kill himself?"). Common examples of this situation include patients with diabetes or hypertension whose conditions respond well to medications while they are in the hospital but are out-of-control on the same regimens at home.

Another "red flag" arises when your patient's illness and disability appear to be far in excess of the evident disease. Take, for example, a patient who asks you to certify his disability to an insurance company because of "high blood pressure and arthritis." From your perspective, his mildly elevated blood pressure is (or ought to be) completely asymptomatic. Similarly, from your perspective, his Heberden's nodes (degenerative osteophytes at the distal interphalangeal joints of his hands) ought also to be asymptomatic. Yet the patient clearly believes that he is unable to work. He may well be disabled, but you must address the personal meaning of his problems to discover why.

A related situation is when the patient has a relatively clear-cut, acute medical problem that resolves (as expected) with treatment, yet symptoms remain. For example, you might learn during an initial interview that your patient was well until his bout of pneumonia 3 months previously. The pneumonia completely resolved with antibiotic therapy, yet the patient has had fatigue, chest pain, and insomnia since then. Alternatively, the patient had an acute myocardial infarction followed by an elective angioplasty several months ago. Although he has not experienced angina or other cardiac-related symptoms, since the hospitalization he has been unable to work.

In some cases you will encounter a situation even more difficult to understand: chronic illness and disability without any identifiable disease. There are a number of common syndromes in medical practice that appear to fit this definition; in some of these, underlying physiologic changes are known (e.g., premenstrual syndrome or late luteal phase disorder), but in others there is no consistent biochemical pattern (e.g., chronic fatigue syndrome, sick building syndrome). Although these patients are undoubtedly ill, the "stuff" of disease is absent or undiscovered. Clearly, the beliefs, values, and expectations of these patients play an important role in their illness experience, both initially and in response to their encounters with health professionals. In some respects these illnesses are similar to **culture-bound syndromes,** characteristic illnesses that originate from and are sustained by an interplay of psychologic and sociocultural factors. Examples of culture-bound syndromes include "susto" in certain Hispanic populations, "ghost sickness" among American Plains Indians, and "neurasthenia," a prevalent disabling ailment in late 19th- and early 20th-century America. Although illnesses like "susto" are readily treated by traditional healers,[4] the orthodox health-care system has found it difficult to incorporate illnesses like chronic fatigue syndrome. We are likely to have culturally defined illnesses in late 20th-century American culture, although they may not be clearly visible to us as such. But you are certain to encounter patients who are sorely disabled, who suffer greatly, and in whom you can discover no physical disease, or in whom physical disease cannot explain the symptoms (see Somatization, p. 193).

ELICITING HEALTH BELIEFS IN THE INTERVIEW

Table 14–2 presents a series of questions you might consider in assessing your patient's beliefs and expectations regarding his or her illness.[5] The use of such questions constitutes a kind of screening test to ascertain whether the patient's beliefs and expectations fall within a "normal" range, a range

TABLE 14-2   QUESTIONS TO ELICIT THE PATIENT'S INTERPRETATION OF THE ILLNESS

Interpretive Level	Examples
Descriptive	How would you describe the problem that concerns you most?
	What are the main difficulties this problem (sickness, illness, disease, or misfortune) has caused for you?
Conceptual	What do you think is wrong, out of balance, or causing your problem?
	What does the illness do to you? How does it work?
	Why did it start when it did?
	What kind of treatment do you think you should receive?
	What are the results you hope for with treatment? Without treatment?
	Apart from me (a medical doctor), who else can help you get better? What else can you do?
Personal	Why did you, as opposed to somebody else, get sick? And get sick now?
	What do you fear most about your sickness?

SOURCE: Adapted from Kleinman A, Eisenberg L, Good B. Culture, illness and care: clinical lessons from anthropological and cross-cultural research. *Ann Intern Med* 1978; 88:251.

in which they will not conflict with medical explanations or treatment, or whether they fall outside this range, in which case they might inhibit you from effectively influencing the patient's behavior[4] unless you utilize them (or, at least, take them into account) in your therapeutic plan.

The first two questions (descriptive level) simply recap what we discussed in Chapter 3 (pp. 50–56) regarding complete characterization of symptoms. It is important to discover precisely what your patient identifies as the major problem for which he or she is seeking help. The ostensible reason for coming, or chief complaint, may not, in fact, be the actual reason for coming. Sometimes it requires probing to get the whole story and to get it straight. The next six questions (conceptual level) address the patient's understanding of the cause, appropriate treatment, and probable outcome of the illness, as well as the premises and logic he or she uses as the basis of those concepts. Because the patient may be aware that his or her beliefs conflict with medical orthodoxy, he or she may not initially feel comfortable explaining them, thinking that you will laugh or become angry. Thus, you must set the stage by developing an empathic connection. The final two questions (personal level) deal with the idiosyncratic personal meaning of symptoms. Here again, mutual respect and trust must be present before patients will express their fears or venture a belief that illness is a punishment for past trangressions.

Here is an example of an elderly woman, blind from glaucoma, who was undergoing chelation therapy, as well as taking standard medical treatment for cerebrovascular and heart disease. Chelation involves the intravenous administration of ethylenediaminetetraacetic acid (EDTA), an agent that binds calcium and other cations, thus removing them from the body when the chelator is excreted in the urine. Chelation is effective in treating lead poisoning, for example, but there is no credible evidence that it removes calcium from atherosclerotic plaques. Moreover, it requires repeated intravenous treatments, which may be dangerous and are definitely expensive. Chelation for atherosclerosis is considered unacceptable medical therapy. This patient has already explained to her new physician that she has been suffering for several months from "creeping numbness" in both legs. This began before her stroke but increased after she recovered from the stroke. Her previous physician evidently did not take this symptom seriously or at least conveyed that impression to the patient. The new physician has helped the patient become comfortable enough to explain her interpretation of the problem and what should be done about it.

Dr: You had this creeping numbness, and they didn't seem to know what to do about it?

Pt: Well, no, and then after the stroke, my back actually . . . I told you about what the doctor said. He said it wasn't important, that it had already happened.

Dr: That your back had already collapsed?

Pt: Well, I didn't understand, I thought that meant my backbones would fall down. But what really happened was, I think, that the muscles that hold the bones together became like stretched out gum bands and, for example, like a car, you drive on an icy road. You want it to go one way and it goes another. I tried to go here but I had no control over my back. No control. I was talking to Dr. Smith about it but he wouldn't do a thing. I mean, it didn't seem to bother him at all. And then my bitter fear for my legs. Then, it actually came to the point where my legs were just like a couple of logs. I would try to sleep at night and turn over and I would drag my legs.

Dr: Is that what made you afraid?

Pt: I was afraid . . . well, I explained to Dr. Smith. "Look, Dr. Smith, there are people that lose the use of their legs and they go and use a wheelchair, but you got to have eyes to guide the wheelchair and I don't have that, so what am I going to do?" But it was like talking to the wall. Once he got very angry. "Do you think that if there would be something that would help you, I wouldn't do it for you?" Well, as if it was a sin for me to be concerned about myself. So anyway, well the situation was really awful, I was really fretting my mind all the time. I just lost the use of my eyes, next I lost the use of my legs, then what to do?

The patient had osteoporosis and vertebral compression fractures. Evidently she had tried first to attribute her leg numbness to the "collapsed" back, but her physician vetoed that explanation and never provided an alternative. Moreover, he seemed to ignore both her symptom and her growing anxiety about it.

Dr: So what did you think, though? I mean, where did the numbness come from?

Pt: Well, then I decided to go to Dr. Brown and he said "I'll chelate you and you'll have no more strokes." So that's when I made up my mind to go to the chelation and I did, and it's better.

Dr: Do you mean Dr. Brown said the numbness was related to the stroke?

Pt: Well, that's the only thing that made sense. Blockage of the arteries. That's what I thought. So chelation must help.

Dr: You were afraid to tell me about this, too, weren't you?

Pt: Yes, because you're not supposed to tell nobody about it.

Dr: Who says you're not supposed to tell?

Pt: Well, you should have seen Dr. Smith. He got mad. I felt so sick that time, he got so mad actually I don't know what was the matter with him. Like he was ready to get a nervous breakdown or something. (Long pause) The thing is, it's so cruel. It's so cruel. Maybe the chelation does do some good, and if it does then why deprive a patient, just because of politics, that's not right. You come to Dr. Brown's office and its always filled with chelating people, you know. So, once I heard this woman telling, not to me, to others, about a friend she knew. How his legs were so bad they turned black and his doctor advised him to have them amputated. Well, that's a horrible prospect! But somebody told him about chelation, so he went and did it, and slowly the color came back in his legs. He started to be okay and he went back to work. This is hard to believe. And when he went to his doctor to show him, the doctor's response was, "If it was up to me I would still amputate." It's hard to believe such extreme cruelty.

Dr: And your legs are better now?

Pt: Yes, well, the numbness is still there, I can notice it, but it's not as bad, really, and I'm not afraid of it.

Dr: How often do you go now?

Pt: Well, in the beginning it's good to go twice a week, but I've never been twice a week. It's not easy sitting 4 hours in one place. It takes 3-1/2 to 4 hours.

Notice that the patient made the assumption that her numbness was due to "blockages" and inferred that chelation would help. Her experience at Dr. Brown's chelation center was quite positive; unlike Dr. Smith, Dr. Brown seemed to know what he was doing. Moreover, she heard a miraculous testimonial of chelation's effectiveness. She also learned that "you shouldn't tell." Had the new physician not made her comfortable and shown interest in her beliefs, he would not have learned that she attributed the problem to calcium deposits ("What do you think is causing your problem?") and sought out chelation ("What kind of treatment do you think you need?"), nor would she have been able to discuss her fears, which arise from the personal level of interpretation ("What do you fear most about your illness?").

The clinician was faced with a patient who had spent much time and money on a form of treatment orthodox medicine considers completely worthless. Earlier physicians had let her down, both by saying there was nothing to be done despite her "bitter fear for my legs," and by becoming angry if she told them about chelation. The main point from this clinician's perspective is that she feels better and her symptoms are largely resolved; no academic discussion of quackery will alter that fact. The questions the clinician will have to ask himself or herself are unrelated to the efficacy of chelation. The important questions are these:

- Are the beliefs really dangerous?
- Do they prohibit medical care that is actually necessary?
- Can I work within the patient's belief system to provide good medical care?

Having answered these, the clinician must take the next step and arrive at a mutually acceptable course of action through the process of negotiation, which we discuss in the next chapter.

S U M M A R Y : Discovering What the Patient Believes

In this chapter we addressed the patient's pre-existing values, beliefs, and expectations regarding illness and health care as they relate to the medical interview. The fact that patients hold nonscientific health beliefs is frequently accepted by health-care professionals who practice in cross-cultural settings. We must recognize, however, that "culture" is not simply an attribute of people who appear to be different from ourselves. The dominant American culture fashions our own beliefs and many of our patients' beliefs about illness. The human experience of illness is never value- or meaning-free. Such beliefs about illness are frequently fragmented and contradictory, rather than being tightly integrated into a coherent system.

Although one's beliefs always influence illness experience, there are a number of "red flags" that suggest that specific attention to health beliefs will contribute greatly to an effective clinical encounter. These include situations in which:

- Chronic illness is poorly controlled despite ostensibly effective treatment
- Illness and disability are disproportional to disease, or acute illness remains symptomatic after disease resolves
- The patient suffers from an illness, but no known disease

In eliciting a patient's interpretation of his or her illness, you may use a series of questions that address the descriptive, conceptual, and personal aspects of these beliefs. Knowledge of these factors is essential for you to understand the effects of serious or chronic illnesses, as well as to promote optimal therapy. In the final chapter, we integrate these concepts into a discussion of negotiation and education in the medical encounter.

References

1. Harwood A. The hot-cold theory of disease. *JAMA* 1971; 216:1153–1158.
2. Snow LF. Folk medical beliefs and their implications for care of patients. *Ann Intern Med* 1974; 81–82.
3. Lipowski ZJ. Physical illness, the individual and the coping process. *Psychiatry Med* 1970; 1: 91–102.
4. Uzzell D. Susto revisited: Illness as strategic role. In: Landy D (ed). *Culture, Disease and Healing*. New York: Macmillan, 1978.
5. Kleinman A, Eisenberg L, Good B. Culture, illness and care: Clinical lessons from anthropological and cross-cultural research. *Ann Intern Med* 1978; 88:251.

Suggested Readings

Good BJ. Culture, diagnosis, and comorbidity. *Cult Med Psychiatry* 1992–1993; 16:427–446.

Jecker NS, Carrese JA, Pearlman RA. Caring for patients in cross-cultural settings. *Hastings Center Rep* 1995; 25:6–14.

Shapiro J, Lenahan P. Family medicine in a culturally diverse world: A solution-oriented approach to common cross-cultural problems in medical encounters. *Fam Med* 1996; 28:249–255.

CHAPTER 15

Not Through Argument but by Contagion

• • •

EDUCATION, INFORMED CONSENT, AND NEGOTIATION

The faith that heals, heals not through argument but by
contagion. But to heal, faith must have substance. A
speculative balance of probability is not enough. The faith that
heals must have deep roots in the personality of the healer.

W. R. Houston, *The Doctor Himself as a Therapeutic Agent*

What are the outcomes of your initial encounter with a patient? What have you achieved when you walk out after completing the history and physical examination? In this book we have emphasized the data collection and hypothesis testing aspects of your medical interview. Your goal in that respect is to achieve the right diagnosis and ultimately to prescribe the right treatment. You then communicate all this to the patient during the termination phase of the interview.

In practice, however, any medical interaction has a more complex outcome than diagnosis alone. When you walk out of the hospital room or the patient walks out of your office, you will have in some way influenced the patient. Of course, you intend to influence the patient's illness through arriving at the correct diagnosis and prescribing appropriate treatment. But you influence patients in at least two other important ways. First, **you influence their behavior** by asking them, for example, to undertake diagnostic studies, follow a regimen of medication, return for follow-up visits, stop smoking, or start exercising. When patients change their behavior in these ways, we say they are "compliant" or that they follow our medical advice. Clearly, the best diagnosis and plan of treatment in the world is useless without this influence on behavior.

Second, **you influence how patients think and feel.** We may cause some change in a patient's concept of what the illness is and what it means and thereby reduce his or her anxiety or, alternatively, increase it. The patient may walk away relieved or sorely distressed. We may have somehow started to diminish his or her burden of suffering, or added to it iatrogenic suffering. It is this sort of influence that Michael Balint had in mind when he taught that "the doctor is the drug."[1]

In other words, your treatment of the patient is not just the medication you prescribe. The drug is just a small part of the influence you may have on the patient and his or her healing process. Even as you complete your initial interview and physical examination, you begin to bring other influences to bear in managing the patient. You may simply be ordering further diagnostic studies while explaining your preliminary findings and expecting the patient to return. Even so, you want to maximize the probability that the patient actually obtains the studies, follows your advice, and returns to your office. You also want to do what you can to make the patient feel better starting today, rather than next week or next month. You want, in some way, if possible, to reduce anxiety and relieve suffering. A skillful medical interview grounded in empathy, respect, and genuineness (see Chap. 2) is the first step in enhancing your patient's active participation in health care and reducing the suffering caused by needless anxiety and uncertainty.

How do you maximize the chance that your influence on the patient will be positive or beneficial? In this book, we have been concerned with the skills of medical interviewing—particularly history taking. Yet, what you do and the way you do it as you take the history will have multiple effects: good technique may maximize the objectivity and precision of the data on which you base your hypotheses, but at the same time good technique may cause the patient to follow your advice and leave your office with a sense of well-being and relief. Sick persons are frequently in a crisis situation when they seek medical help, a time when seemingly small interventions have significant outcomes. Among all these possible outcomes, relevant ones cluster

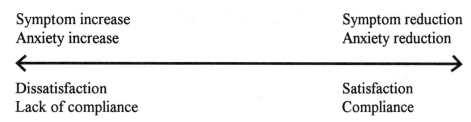

Symptom increase   Symptom reduction
Anxiety increase   Anxiety reduction

Dissatisfaction   Satisfaction
Lack of compliance   Compliance

FIGURE 15–1. Possible outcomes of the medical interaction.

into beneficial or harmful groups, as shown in Figure 15–1. In other words, **any doctor-patient interaction is likely to influence the suffering of a sick person.**

Most treatment in medicine requires active patient cooperation. Except for comatose patients, who receive their intravenous fluids and medications with little, if any, compliance necessary on their part, it is difficult to imagine a medical care situation in which the behavioral component of therapy is not significant. Although "compliance" is a common term in medical parlance, it has two drawbacks. First, the term suggests that the physician's orders are uniquely right and that any patient who fails to be 100 percent compliant will have an outcome that will be less than successful. Second, the term suggests a passive, "plastic" patient rather than an active, participating one. To some extent, the word "adherence" does not share the second connotation, but it still contains the first. The patient must adhere, albeit actively, to the doctor's correct regimen. Rather than using these terms, we prefer to talk simply about the patient's behavior with regard to treatment and instructions and to consider how much the clinician himself or herself influences that behavior.

This chapter deals with how clinicians influence patients in the course of everyday clinician-patient interactions. We show how these interactions are learning experiences that can be used to encourage personal responsibility and behavioral change. In Chapter 9 we presented some simple steps to enhance patient understanding in the office and avoid the patient's perception that "the doctor doesn't explain anything," as well as the physician's perception that "the patient doesn't understand" (see Table 9–3). In this chapter we share some theories about what works in conveying information not only with regard to "instructing" patients but also with regard to establishing appropriate expectations about the illness and its treatment, an important component not only of adherence but also of informed consent and malpractice prevention. Finally, we consider the art of negotiation and its component skills and behaviors.

EDUCATION: CONVEYING THE INFORMATION

Why don't patients always follow their doctors' instructions? A number of hypotheses have been suggested to explain so-called noncompliant behavior[2]:

- The **personality hypothesis,** which holds that something in the patient's basic personality structure interferes
- The **psychodynamic hypothesis,** which holds that some important defense mechanism, such as denial, prevents compliance
- The **interpersonal hypothesis,** in which affective problems arising from the doctor-patient interaction prevent full compliance
- The **cognitive hypothesis,** which holds that the problem has to do with communication per se—words and concepts—and the simple recall of what the clinician said

Although each of these must play a part at least some of the time, many studies have demonstrated that patients simply do not remember a good deal of what is said to them. They cannot do what is recommended if they fail to remember what medication to take or how to take it. (Investigators agree that patients, on average, immediately remember 50 to 60 percent of the information doctors give them, and about 45 to 55 percent several weeks later.[2,3]) Interestingly, neither the intelligence nor age of the patient seem to be important factors in how much is remembered. Even writing down the information, which on the surface would appear to be a fail-safe method, does not, in fact, necessarily lead to a better outcome in terms of better compliance or the amount of information remembered. Of note, patients who have a moderate level of anxiety about their problems are more likely to remember than if they have either very high (paralyzing and distracting) or very low (nonmotivating) anxiety levels. So the first step in ensuring patient involvement, conceptually at least, is to make sure that the patient understands what you are saying and remembers it. How do you do that? Consider the following example:

Dr: So we're going to treat your hypertension with this diuretic and . . .

Pt: My hyperTENSION? But I don't feel tense . . .

Dr: . . . We'll see how things go and we'll keep adding drugs until we get things in control.

Pt: I don't know, with my job and all, I can't afford not to be sharp . . .

This example is not unlike the one presented in Chapter 9 (p. 167), and it is easy to see the clinician's errors. Not only the words but the style of this segment of the interaction suggest a range of behaviors and missed opportunities. We are left wondering whether the clinician, who must have taken the patient's blood pressure (we hope several times) during the interaction, has been silent all this time, thereby raising the patient's anxiety by saying nothing until the very end about the patient's blood pressure, then using the word "hypertension" which seems common enough but can be misundertsood by even the most well-educated patient. The clinician seems to be rushing right to a discussion of treatment before even explaining the diagnosis and goes on to be vague about what the patient can expect, thereby increasing uncertainty (and anxiety). Note, too, that the use of the word "drug" in the context of the word "hyperTENSION" appears to leave this high-powered attorney totally confused (not a state that he or anyone else is likely to enjoy). The clinician needs, instead, to facilitate understanding with the following behaviors:

- Use words and phrases more likely to be understood by the patient (words such as "red" and "high blood pressure" work just as well as "erythematous" and "hypertension").
- Be concrete and specific about the problems being considered and what the patient can expect.
- Inquire about how much the patient understands and give feedback about that understanding.
- Encourage questions.

In summary, rather than instructing the patient, here is how the same clinician might, on a better day, share her findings and arrive at a plan with the patient:

Dr: Well, as I mentioned during my exam, when I take your blood pressure it is repeatedly high.

Pt: Yeah, you said that and it's making me kinda worried.

Dr: Well, we consider normal anything under 140 over 90 (writing out and showing the patient), and yours is 160 over 105.

Pt: Uh huh, umm.

Dr: Another word for high blood pressure is "hypertension," even though it has nothing necessarily to do with tension or feeling tense. What I'd like to do next is explain to you what this means, what we should do about it, and give you time to ask questions so I'm sure you understand. Okay?

This time the doctor has done a number of things to influence the patient by better transfer of information. The patient may well be more satisfied than in our first example and go home less anxious and confused about his condition. In addition, the doctor also anticipated common errors in patient understanding ("it has nothing to do with tension"), not only laying the groundwork for the proposed plan of treatment but also making it easier for the patient to reveal other possible misconceptions.

INFORMED CONSENT

Once we have conveyed the basic information and our recommendations, we must be sure that the patient understands and agrees to the plan. When patients answer our questions during the interview, submit to a physical examination, and allow themselves to be stuck by needles or penetrated by x-rays, they give implied consent (what we have earlier termed a "contract") by their actions. More invasive procedures and specialized therapies have sufficient potential risk that patients must explicitly consent to them on the basis of adequate information about benefits, risks, and alternatives. In this chapter we cannot examine fully the moral and legal doctrine of informed consent or the controversies about whether (and how much) informed consent is possible in medical practice. Nevertheless, you often will be required to obtain explicit consent. How do you obtain consent? What do you explain? The following guidelines should be of some help.

The Process

Informed consent is a process, not a form or piece of paper. Standard consent forms contain bureaucratic language and require the patient's (and a witness's) signature. You can use such a form as an outline to guide discussion, but the patient's act of signing this paper does not constitute informed consent. And, though it does serve as evidence, the signed consent form is not necessarily sufficient proof of informed consent in court. The legal doctrine of informed consent demands four elements in the consent process, shown in Table 15–1. Because informed consent is a process, it requires skillful patient-doctor interaction. Katz[4] employs the metaphor of conversation to describe informed consent. Although there are ordinarily no strict rules to determine when a conversation is finished, "most people have a good intuitive grasp of what it means for a conversation to be finished, what it means to change the subject in the middle of a conversation, and what it means to later reopen a conversation one had thought was completed when something new has just arisen." Similarly, in everyday practice we often know when a competent patient has voluntarily and with understanding agreed to a diagnostic study or treatment. Brody[5] suggests what he calls the "transparency" standard of consent for everyday medical practice. According to this standard, adequate informed consent is obtained when a reasonably informed patient is allowed to participate in the medical decision to the extent that the patient wishes. In turn, "reasonably informed" consists of two fea-

TABLE 15–1 ELEMENTS OF INFORMED CONSENT

Informed

Information: The patient should be provided with information that a "reasonable person" would want to know about the nature of the procedure, benefits, risks, and alternative courses of action.

Understanding: The patient must understand the information provided.

Consent

Voluntary: The patient's decision must be freely made, without evidence of coercion.

Competency: The patient should be capable of making an autonomous medical decision in this particular setting.

tures: (1) the physician discloses the basis on which the proposed treatment, or alternative possible treatments, have been chosen; and (2) the patient is allowed to ask questions suggested by the disclosure of the physician's reasoning, and those questions are answered to the patient's satisfaction.[5] In other words, the clinician reveals his or her thought process so that it is transparent to the patient and then encourages those good old open-ended questions, which form the basis of the best medical interviews (see Chap. 3). In our example the clinician might go on to say:

> **Dr:** I know you're concerned about your blood pressure, so let me tell you what I'm thinking. We know we can reduce the risk to your health by treating your blood pressure, and we know that there are a number of very safe and effective medicines that have been used for many years. So here's what I'd like to recommend. . . . What do you think about that?

The important issue here is that consent must be obtained in the context of a conversation during which clear explanations are given and questions are answered, and the patient's competence and understanding are assessed. Although we often think of informed consent only in the context of explaining risky procedures, it is a part of the most ordinary patient interactions. Such a conversation may lead to negotiation and compromise (as we discuss later) if the patient objects to proposed procedures or treatments; and the conversation is usually one that has the potential to be reopened at a later time. The therapeutic core qualities of empathy, genuineness, and respect (see Chap. 2) build trust and thereby facilitate the consent process, an important component of malpractice suit prevention, especially when the uncertainty of the outcome is explored. In the words of Gutheil and coworkers,[6] informed consent is an "interaction between physician and patient, a dialogue intended not only to satisfy a legal requirement but to do more as well. The real clinical opportunity offered by informed consent is that of transforming uncertainty from a threat to the doctor-patient alliance into the very basis upon which an alliance can be formed. . . . Note that our approach stresses the selection of what to say to patients rather than such advice as taking more time with patients or telling them more. In practice, less time is taken and more is understood: sound efficiency of communication, not mere volume of words, is the desideratum."[6]

Barriers

In practice, there are often **barriers** to informed consent that do not arise simply from patient ignorance or physician noncooperation. These barriers (Table 15–2) inhibit strict adherence to the elements of informed consent.[7,8] One problem is that some patients think decision making ought to be in the hands of their physicians and defer to their physicians' judgments. They opt out of the formal decision. Nonetheless, most patients desire to be thoroughly informed about what is going on. Caregivers should not confuse ready acceptance of a diagnostic test with disinterest in its purpose and characteristics. Another problem is that the medical care process often confuses patients because there are many decisions to be made, the decisions occur at different times, and frequently a variety of people are responsible. It is difficult to focus on one decision or one issue. You have an excellent opportunity to help your patients by listening to their concerns and by encouraging and then answering their questions.

TABLE 15–2 BARRIERS TO INFORMED CONSENT

Nature of Medical Decisions

Treatment decisions tend to evolve over time, rather than being quick and clear.

Often numerous, related decisions must be made.

The decision-making process often involves numerous people.

Patient Characteristics

The patient wants information but believes the actual decision is the doctor's task.

The patient does not know which doctor is responsible.

The patient fails to "hear" because of conflict or denial.

Physician Characteristics

Doctors do not understand the rationale for patient involvement.

Doctors do not take time to explain issues clearly to the patient.

SOURCE: Based on Lidz, CW, et al.[7]

Evaluating Competence in the Interview

Competence is a legal concept, not a medical one. Formal adjudication of competence can only occur in court. The physician's role is to gather relevant information and to decide whether a patient's competence should be called into question. What clinical information is relevant to this question?

Some physicians think that a patient's refusal of medically indicated care is in itself evidence of incompetence. This might be called an **outcome standard**. It means that if a patient's decision is the medically appropriate one (the right outcome, from our point of view), we presume the patient is competent. If the decision is medically inappropriate, we suspect incompetence. The issue of competency rarely arises if the patient agrees to the lumbar puncture or to the cardiac catheterization; it is only when the patient refuses the interventions that we wonder about his or her competence. By this definition, every person who refuses aggressive treatment might have his or her wishes overruled by well-meaning, paternalistic doctors. Although we should, in fact, discuss issues thoroughly and make careful observations (i.e., mental status) when patients refuse what seems to us to be clearly beneficial care, the fact of refusal is not in itself evidence for incompetence.

The President's Commission on Ethical Decisions in Medical and Health Care suggests that we use information about the patient's **process of decision making**, rather than relying solely on information about potential outcome or patient status. Such a standard further requires that we look at the patient's decision-making process as it relates to the issue at hand, rather than relying on more global observations, such as the patient's pattern of forgetfulness or eccentricities, or the fact that the patient is sometimes incontinent or confused. Just as the concept of transparency requires that patients be able to see our thinking process, the issue of competency requires that we see theirs. What specific observations are required to apply a decision-making standard of competency?

Appelbaum and Grisso[9] suggest four criteria commonly accepted by the courts:

- The patient must be able to communicate a choice.
- The patient must be able to understand information about a treatment decision.
- The patient must appreciate the medical situation and its consequences. This means awareness of illness and the relative likelihood of various outcomes, given various treatment options.
- The patient must be able to use logical processes to evaluate information and compare options.

It is crucial here to distinguish between a logical process and a correct or reasonable conclusion. As discussed in Chapter 14, a patient's beliefs or values might be different from those of most people, and using those beliefs as premises, the patient might reach a perfectly logical conclusion that is clearly wrong from *our* point of view. For example, Christian Scientists believe that illness is illusory and represents an error in thinking that can be corrected by study and prayer; they may logically conclude that medical treatments are not in their best interests because such treatments are based on the alternate belief that sickness is real.

The relevant data required to apply criteria for competence all arise from a careful and compassionate patient-doctor conversation. Inability to communicate a choice is usually obvious if it is caused by decreased consciousness or psychotic thought disorder. However, extreme ambivalence may lead a patient to switch his or her decision abruptly several times during a short period. Impairments of attention span, memory, and intelligence, as well as thought disorders, may interfere with the ability to understand information and to appreciate consequences of the medical situation. These can be assessed during the routine mental status part of your interview. Assessing the capacity to reason logically is more subtle, and some courts have considered logical handling of data to be too strong a criterion to require as evidence of competency. Psychiatric consultation is sometimes necessary to assist in this assessment. In any case, an understanding of the patient's beliefs and value system is required to understand his or her reasoning about medical decisions.

Sometimes patient refusal of indicated tests or treatment can be frustrating, even anger provoking. Respect for the patient, however, demands that we be very cautious about questioning a patient's competence in order to act against his or her wishes. Here are some guidelines that might be helpful in developing your own thinking about competence in medical care decisions:

- A patient's refusal of the best medical option is not in itself evidence of incompetence; likewise, acceptance of the best medical option is not in itself evidence of competence.

- Presence of psychiatric symptoms or an identified psychiatric disorder does not in itself mean the patient is incompetent. Many severely ill patients are depressed, but depression does not necessarily impair decision-making ability (at least not to the extent that it threatens competence).

- Decisions about medical care are essentially value decisions and are determined by religious, cultural, and personal beliefs, not biomedical factors alone.

- Physicians are experts about their patients' medical best interests but not necessarily about their best interests in general. Patients may have a more global view of their welfare, based on religious, cultural, or other values.

Once the patient understands the problem, what happens when, in the course of eliciting the patient's informed consent, you discover a lack of agreement about what should happen? Clinician and patient must take the next step and arrive at a mutually acceptable course of action through the process of negotiation, which we discuss now.

NEGOTIATION

Although patients cannot follow your advice unless they understand and remember it, patients may also fail to follow advice if they do not agree with or consent to it. So it is necessary to learn what the patient believes needs to be done for the illness. You can use this information to help the patient get well by attempting to change the patient's beliefs, by altering your therapeutic plan to accommodate them, or by reaching some intermediate, negotiated, therapeutic alliance. **Negotiation** is a process in which people use discussion and compromise to arrive at a settlement of some issue. In practice, negotiation is a way of optimizing patient compliance and understanding and is a sign of respect for the patient. Once you have spoken with the patient and performed a physical examination, you will have some hypotheses about the patient's illness, although you may remain uncertain about why the patient is ill or what the natural course of the illness will be. You will want to influence the patient's behavior, decrease his or her anxiety, and give the patient a better sense of control over the problem. How do you do this in the clinical interview?

With the theme of mutual participation, let us look at crucial aspects of negotiation in medical practice[10,11]:

- A respectful atmosphere that puts the patient at ease
- A method of ascertaining the patient's goals and expectations
- A positive attitude
- Education for the patient about the problem and its treatment
- A process of eliciting suggestions, preferences, and disagreements from the patient
- An adequate response to the patient's concerns, particularly in terms of feelings
- The ability to reach a compromise position, when there is conflict, by a good-faith "give-and-take"

This mutual-participation model of doctor-patient interaction assumes four subject areas[12]:

- Agreement on what the clinical information really is
- Agreement on the nature of the problem

- Agreement about what can or should be done
- Consent for procedures or treatments

The characteristics of your patient, your traits, and the qualities of the relationship between you may facilitate or hinder compliance. In the context of negotiation, it is important to understand the patient's comprehension, decision-making processes, and environment, as well as remembering that "acceptance of the diagnosis is particularly important because of the frequent occurrence of erroneous powerful health beliefs."[13] Certain things you do within the interview in turn influence the patient's behavior:

- Eliciting and respecting the patient's concerns, where both the patient and physician communicate their preferences
- Evaluating the patient's comprehension and educating him or her in order to prevent the part of noncompliance that may be "nonvoluntary"
- Learning about the patient's specific health beliefs, particularly those regarding perceived susceptibility and perceived severity
- Understanding the patient's perception of trade-offs between benefits and risks, and between the quality and quantity of life

These guidelines restate in different terms the familiar themes of empathy, respect, communication skills, and acknowledgment of the patient's beliefs and expectations. You influence patients more when you respect them, communicate well with them, and understand "where they're coming from." An additional theme is that of uncertainty. The question of uncertainty is particularly important to emphasize for those just learning how to interview patients and negotiate with them. The uncertainty that you experience is only partially because you are a beginner; much uncertainty is intrinsic to interactions between health-care professionals and patients. From this perspective, you are negotiating not only to make the patient more likely to follow your suggestions or to understand your formulation, but also to achieve a better healing effect than could be obtained from a unilateral decision on your part combined with 100 percent patient compliance. This means that negotiation requires sharing your uncertainty with the patient.

We summarize the components of negotiation in Table 15–3 and end this chapter with the following case example, which demonstrates the interactive nature of clinical problem solving and the negotiation that occurs as new data are added. The case illustrates negotiation both in the "give-and-take" bargaining and the "maneuver to find a path" senses of the word.

A 25-year-old woman came to her doctor's office with the complaint of a severe and persistent vaginal itch. She expressed her distress and sum-

TABLE 15-3 COMPONENTS OF NEGOTIATION

1. Respect the patient and deal with feelings.
2. Inform the patient (i.e., using understandable terms, present, verify, and interpret the evidence with regard to diagnosis and therapy).
3. Elicit the patient's goals. (What would you like to happen? What do you think will happen?)

   Elicit the patient's suggestions. (How do you think we should handle this? What do you think is wrong?)

   Elicit the patient's preferences. (Do you prefer medical therapy for this problem, or do you think surgery might work better for you?)
4. Help the patient weigh risks and benefits, including trade-offs between the quality and quantity of life.
5. Formulate an agreement on the nature of the problem and a plan of action.

marized her problem in the opening statement that we encountered previously in Chapter 3 (p. 57):

Pt: Well, I have a terrible vaginal itch, and I don't know whether it's from vaginitis or whether it's the urinary tract infection—you know—ah, my regular doctor treated me for vaginitis first . . .

Dr: That was Doctor X?

Pt: Uh huh, then I, um, got a urinary tract infection, then the vaginitis came back, but during the whole ordeal I've never got no relief.

We learn several important things about this patient from her opening statement: she is suffering ("terrible," "ordeal," "no relief"), she is medically sophisticated ("vaginitis," "urinary tract infection"), and she is not well educated in the sense of formal schooling ("I've never got no . . . ").

The physician performs an examination, then leaves the room to examine a specimen of vaginal secretions under the microscope, returning with the news that the infection is clearly caused by *Trichomonas vaginalis* and can be easily and effectively treated with a single dose of eight pills. At this point, both patient and physician agree on the nature of the problem: it is a *Trichomonas* infection. To the patient, the end of her suffering is in sight. The physician begins to write out a prescription. But, seeing the name of the drug as the physician writes it, the patient makes an unexpected comment:

Pt: Flagyl. You don't have any . . . there's nothing else you can take besides Flagyl, huh?

Up until this point, it would appear as though the physician has made not only an accurate diagnosis but also a correct decision about therapy, with which the patient will be happy. But the patient, instead of being appropriately grateful for the physician's expertise, is not satisfied. The negotiation begins.

Dr: It's the best for it.
Pt: Okay, but I might . . . well, I'll try it.

You could imagine a scenario here in which the physician simply says "fine," and the patient is left to her own doubts about the drug, perhaps taking it, perhaps not. But the physician, listening to her hesitation, replies:

Dr: What's the problem?
Pt: But I think I was allergic to that.
Dr: Why do you think that?
Pt: Because I remember taking Flagyl before, and it did something . . . I think I broke out in hives or something.
Dr: Really?
Pt: But I'll try it. If I break out I'll let you know, but I think I did.
Dr: That's a worry . . . let me look at the record. It says here that you were sensitive to ampicillin and sulfa . . . now could it have been . . . Oh, it does say Flagyl . . .
Pt: I think it was just hives. Maybe I've outgrown it.
Dr: I don't want you to take it if you had hives from it.
Pt: Well, maybe I'll have . . . I'll have outgrown it 'cause I think it's been a while back.
Dr: (Still looking through the chart) Yeah, it does say Flagyl.

The patient actually begins with an interpretation ("allergic") of some past event associated with the drug. Physician and patient then exchange information, together trying to verify or refute that interpretation. The patient provides supporting evidence with the descriptive term "hives," while the physician searches for other evidence by going through the patient's chart. (She is new to this physician but had previously been seen in the same clinic.) However, this is more than a simple discussion of evidence, as we can see both patient ("I'll try it") and physician ("I don't want you to take it . . . ") apparently on the verge of decisions, albeit opposite ones. Perhaps, seeing the physician's concern and despite her willingness to risk hives, the patient offers a new interpretation to the data ("Maybe I'll have outgrown it"). The physician then offers:

Dr: What we could do is we could treat your husband and we could treat you with something else, but . . .
Pt: Well, if that's the best, I want that.
Dr: . . . most of the "something elses" aren't as effective.
Pt: Well, I'll take Flagyl. It can only break me out in hives a day like . . . it'll probably go away in the morning.
Dr: I would be kind of worried about that before prescribing it for you because you could get an even more serious reaction to it.

Data have been exchanged ("I was allergic"), verified ("hives," written record), and now reinterpreted ("I've outgrown it"). The patient, echoing the physician's "it's the best," rejects the notion of "something else" by reversing the implication of concession in her earlier statement on taking Flagyl ("well, I'll try it"). In the context of the physician's earlier statement, "something else" would have to be seen as decidedly inferior. We are tiptoeing on a threshold-of-risk boundary: Take Flagyl and get rid of the itch but risk an allergic reaction, or take something else and avoid the reaction but risk not curing the itch. Much of what the patient says in subsequent statements suggests that she places a higher value on getting rid of the itch than on avoiding an allergic reaction. The patient acknowledges that there is a risk involved but discounts it ("just hives"); the physician, on the other hand, emphasizes that the risk is more than that characterized by the patient ("you could get an even more serious reaction").

The decision has become problematic, and we begin to see patient and physician engage in a dialogue regarding risks and benefits. Lacking the data necessary to value or weigh the risks, the physician returns to a discussion of the evidence, by turning again to the written record to find the supporting data for the diagnosis of allergy, while the patient in turn supplies additional details pointedly aimed at discrediting her own report of an allergic reaction:

Dr: Uh, let me see what Dr. X said about that.
Pt: I don't even think that Dr. X was here when I had that.
Dr: Dr. Y? Dr. Z? . . . because that may be why you've been treated with all this other stuff.
Pt: But they, I remember I told them it did that to me, it might notta been that.
Dr: But it does say you're allergic to it.
Pt: That's cause I told him that.

Dr: I've never heard of anybody being allergic to it but it's . . .
Pt: That's what I'm saying, it's . . .
Dr: . . . certainly possible.
Pt: Probably what happened was I broke out in hives in reaction to other things.

It is remarkable that the patient understands that the source of the data in question—or rather the interpretation in question—is herself ("cause I told him that") and that she may not be the most reliable interpreter of the evidence. Perhaps, if she is the source of the original interpretation, she can also be the source of a new interpretation. In the end the physician is persuaded—to some extent. Note the ensuing discussion in which various outcomes are valued and a decision is reached:

Dr: Well, I'll tell you what I want you to do. Since you have taken a lot of drugs because of all these urinary infections . . .
Pt: That might be why it's never left.
Dr: Uh hum . . .
Pt: So I'd rather take the Flagyl.
Dr: Well I'll tell you what I want you to do.
Pt: . . . it won't be your fault . . .
Dr: Well, I'm still the one that prescribes it. Let me tell you what I'd like you to do. I'd like you to take one pill out of your eight as a test dose. OK? And if you have no reaction to it, then we will hope it is safe to take the rest, though we can't know for sure.
Pt: Um hmm.
Dr: Today, just one, see what happens, and if you have no reaction to it at all, then tomorrow take the remaining seven and have your husband take his eight. OK?
Pt: OK.
Dr: OK? So if you are allergic we'll know.
Pt: Yeah, I'll get hives (ha ha).
Dr: Well, let's just be on the safe side, let's use a test dose . . . OK? Because *Trichomonas*, while it's uncomfortable, it can't kill you, so you know . . .
Pt: It can drive you mad.
Dr: I know, but the point is that we don't want to do anything that would be harmful to your health.

Although there was a lot of back-and-forth maneuvering, the physician takes ultimate responsibility for the decision ("I'm still the one that prescribes it"), but the decision is clearly influenced by the value the patient places on getting rid of the itch ("It can drive you mad"). The patient took the medication, had no reaction, and got rid of the itch. It is not difficult to imagine a different situation with a patient who, perhaps, had suffered more from hives. In that case, the negotiation would have resulted in a different outcome, such as the prescribing of a somewhat less effective therapy.

S U M M A R Y : Influencing the Patient

In this chapter we have addressed the question of how you **influence** the patient's behavior and feelings through the clinical interview. We have divided this influencing skill into components for the sake of discussion, although in practice they often flow together. First, the patient's **understanding** and **recall** of information must serve as a basis for any behavioral influence we might have. The patient cannot cooperate unless he or she knows what to do and how to do it. Moreover, the patient is not likely to be motivated to cooperate unless he or she knows why something is to be done and how it works. Second, the patient must agree **voluntarily** to the proposed plan, in a process known as **informed consent**. Finally, we discussed the role of **negotiation** in achieving an effective therapeutic outcome. Respect for the patient and knowledge of his or her beliefs would not necessarily help you to influence the patient unless you can use these while engaging in a process of negotiation, the **give-and-take of ideas and feelings that allows you to arrive at a mutually agreed-upon plan of action.**

References

1. Balint M. *The Doctor and His Patient and the Illness*. New York, International Universities Press, 1972.
2. Ley P. Toward better doctor-patient communication. Contributions from social and experimental psychology. In: Bennett AE. (Ed.) *Communication Between Doctors and Patients*. Oxford, Nuffield Provincial Hospitals Trust, Oxford University Press, 1976, pp. 77–98.
3. Johnson PE, Duran AS, Hassebrock F, et al. Expertise and error in diagnostic reasoning. *Cognitive Science* 1981; 5:235–283.
4. Katz J. *The Silent World of Doctor and Patient*. New York, The Free Press, 1984.
5. Brody H. Transparency: Informed consent in primary care. *Hastings Cent Rep* 1989; 19:5–9.
6. Gutheil TG, Bursztajn H, Brodsky A. Malpractice prevention through the sharing of uncertainty. Informed consent and the therapeutic alliance. *N Engl J Med* 1984; 311:49.
7. Lidz CW, et al. Barriers to informed consent. *Ann Intern Med* 1983; 99:539–543.
8. Lidz CW, et al. *Informed Consent: A Study of Psychiatric Decision Making*. New York, Guilford Press, 1983.
9. Appelbaum PS, Grisso T. Assessing patients' capacities to consent to treatment. *N Engl J Med* 1988; 319:1635–1638.
10. Bernarde MA, Mayerson EW. Patient-physician negotiation. *JAMA* 1978; 239:1413.

11. Beckman HB, Frankel RM. The effect of physician behavior on the collection of data. *Ann Intern Med* 1984; 101:692–696.
12. Heaton PB. Negotiations as an integral part of the physician's clinical reasoning. *J Fam Pract* 1981; 13:845.
13. Eraker SA, Politser P. How decisions are reached: Physician and patient. *Ann Intern Med* 1982; 97:262.

Suggested Readings

Redelmeier DA, Rozin P, Kahneman D. Understanding patients' decisions. *JAMA* 1993; 270:72–76.

Sackett DL, Haynes RB. *Compliance With Therapeutic Regimens*. Baltimore, Johns Hopkins University Press, 1976.

Index

• • •

An "f" following a page number indicates a figure; a "t" indicates a table.